This is a very easy book to read. Full of delightful insights and excitement at the birth of the authors' first child, many expectant parents will connect with it. The inclusion of stories from other couples means that this is more than the simple journey of one young couple becoming parents for the first time.

*Lindsay and Mark Melluish, authors and pioneeers of the Family Time Parenting Children Course*

Will and Louie are a thoughtful, sensitive and prayerful couple. Their insights into impending parenthood will be helpful to anyone expecting a child.

*Frog and Amy Orr-Ewing, authors and speakers*

Full of practical, down-to-earth advice and fresh biblical insights, Will and Louie reflect on their experience as first-time parents going through pregnancy, childbirth and early parenthood. Sharing their own stories with warmth and transparency, they offer a great resource to new parents embarking on this great new adventure!

*Revd Chris Saxton, vicar of American Lutheran Church in Phoenix, Arizona, and Jo Saxton, 3D Ministries, author and speaker*

Will & Lucinda
van der Hart

# The
# Pregnancy
# Book

Spiritual & emotional survival
for first-time parents

Foreword by Nicky and Sila Lee

ivp

INTER-VARSITY PRESS
Norton Street, Nottingham NG7 3HR, England
*Email: ivp@ivpbooks.com*
*Website: www.ivpbooks.com*

*First published 2010*

**British Library Cataloguing in Publication Data**
A catalogue record for this book is available from the British Library.

ISBN: 978-1-84474-440-4

Set in Monotype Dante 12/15pt
Typeset in Great Britain by Servis Filmsetting Ltd, Stockport, Cheshire
Printed and bound in Great Britain by Ashford Colour Press Ltd, Gosport,
Hampshire

To Skye,
without whom this book would never have been written

# CONTENTS

# FOREWORD

This book fills a vital gap left by other books on pregnancy and parenting. *The Pregnancy Book* is far more than information. It is about challenging and changing the way we think. It is both spiritual and down to earth. Will and Louie tell not only their own personal, and sometimes very different, stories about the journey towards becoming a father and a mother, but they show just how flexible we need to be to meet the demands of parenthood. They help new parents to understand how life changes forever, and that having a baby takes us beyond the ability to control every aspect of our lives to a greater dependence on God.

*The Pregnancy Book* provides an opportunity for parents and prospective parents to take stock of the way their emotional and spiritual well-being will affect their parenting, and to address those issues that arise. As parents we can all too easily either imitate or react against the way we ourselves were brought up. By helping us to recognize the effects of our own upbringing, they enable us to make real choices about the ways in which we want to parent.

While Will and Louie's reflections on the pregnancy and birth of their first child are always fascinating and sometimes hilarious, this book is not based solely on their experiences. As well as telling the stories of other parents today, they also explore the accounts of pregnancies and births in the Bible, and draw out lessons to inspire and encourage their readers.

Through the authors' sharing of their own journey of

faith, pregnancy and parenthood, this valuable and easy-to-read book will help many others to become more effective and more fulfilled parents.

Nicky and Sila Lee
Authors of *The Marriage Book* and *The Parenting Book*
January 2010

# ACKNOWLEDGMENTS

We would like to thank IVP for their support over the last year, and in particular our editor Eleanor Trotter. *The Pregnancy Book* represents the stories of scores of different parents in the early phase of life with a new child, and we are very grateful to everyone who offered us an opinion, anecdote or testimony about pregnancy and parenthood. We also want to thank our wonderful church, who have loved us and built us up throughout our journey into parenthood.

We are so grateful to our parents for encouraging us as we've put our thoughts on paper, and for providing some 'grandparent time' so that we could sit down and write. Finally, we thank our daughter Skye for showing us the way when we didn't have a clue what to do! We pray that you will agree with what we have written when you are old enough to read it.

Will and Lucinda van der Hart

# INTRODUCTION

## By Louie

'Having a baby will change your life. Get ready! Your whole world is about to be turned upside down.'

Are those words familiar? Hearing them from more experienced parents time and time again during my pregnancy made me edgy about what was coming my way. It felt like a conspiracy theory – everyone tells you that something is about to rock your world, but nobody will say how.

Like every parent-to-be, my dream was to be the best parent I could be. But as my pregnancy progressed, I began to wonder what I could do to prepare for bringing a child into the world. How could I give this little person the best possible start in life? Our culture told me: hit the shops and buy all the top-of-the-range stuff, then absorb your preferred parenting expert's advice and get ready to follow it to the letter.

Somehow this approach seemed too practical and simplistic. I was hungry for some sound Christian wisdom on this strange new experience that was pregnancy and what it meant to become a parent. How on earth would I make the shift from being childless to being a human with responsibility for nurturing a new life?

Becoming a parent affects a person on every level: physically, mentally, emotionally, relationally and spiritually. This book will help you prepare for, and work through, those changes. It is not a book about dealing with the physiological transformation brought on by pregnancy, or a practical guide to caring for a newborn baby. Instead, here we consider pregnancy as God's chosen time for us to prepare holistically for becoming parents.

Will and I co-wrote this book through my pregnancy and the first year of our daughter Skye's life. We are certainly not parenting experts, however. We have a lot to learn, and I sometimes wonder whether we'll look back in a few years' time and have developed a completely new set of opinions from the ones expressed here. But even if that's the case, the thoughts you read in this book were live for us during pregnancy and the very early stages of parenthood. I hope that this is what gives them value. Here is our honest, messy attempt at launching into parenthood with God's help, recorded between the hospital checks, baby feeds and nappy changes.

Gaining insight into what may lie ahead can be a helpful part of preparing for parenthood. With this in mind, towards the end of the book we explore some of the issues we have worked through as new parents. As you read, you will also find that we share the thoughts and stories of other parents-to-be and new parents. These are included to give you a peek into the world of a new parent, and to offer some perspectives other than our own. We are very grateful to all our friends who have allowed us to use their personal stories. To avoid embarrassment and indiscretion, we have used some composite stories and changed some names.

Becoming a parent is not always a straightforward process. Maybe you struggled to conceive, had to deal with the trauma of miscarriage or find yourself in the midst of a pregnancy with complications. None of us is immune to such things, and while this book doesn't focus primarily on complications in pregnancy or the many ethical issues that surround conception, I hope you will find it sensitive to them.

Equally you may be stepping into parenthood alone. While as Christians we often emphasize the importance of a loving, committed marriage as the ideal context for starting a family, remember that in the New Testament Mary herself was unmarried when she got pregnant. I have met countless single parents who are doing the most incredible job of raising their children. If you are reading this as a parent-to-be who will be going it alone, some of the challenges you will face will be different from those starting out on this road as a married couple. I hope you will still find much of what you read here relevant and helpful.

Finally, a word for those of you who feel it is out of character to read a book on becoming a parent. Perhaps, like me, you don't naturally melt into a gooey heap over a little child. Perhaps you haven't dreamt of being a mother (or father) since you were ten. Maybe you get nervous when you hold a baby (and until I had my own, I did too). Or it may be that your pregnancy has been awaited, prayed about and longed for over a period of months or even years. The elation you are experiencing may not have been paralleled by anything that has previously happened in your life. Perhaps you are reading, not as a first-time parent, but as someone who already has a child and who wants to do things differently the second time around.

Whatever place you are in, be assured it is OK. Becoming a parent is all about trusting God to get us to where he needs us to be in order to bring up children his way. Every parent-to-be starts the pregnancy journey in a place of inexperience and vulnerability. However you feel, parenthood is a calling. Praise God that he promises to equip those whom he calls!

Will and I hope and pray that you will engage with this time of preparation and launch confidently into parenthood. We want you not only to survive as new parents, but to thrive in your new role. God will give you everything you need for the journey. We pray that he will teach you how to become the parent he made you to be, and that on the way you'll enjoy exciting new glimpses of the first, original and most loving Parent ever.

Lucinda van der Hart (also known as Louie)

# PART I: PREGNANCY

## 1. HOW DO YOU HOLD A BABY?
### BEGINNING THE PREGNANCY JOURNEY

**By Louie**

I felt like a fraud organizing a baby shower. I'd only previously ever been to one of these cupcake-and-cute-baby-outfit-fuelled events before, and I knew nothing about babies. But Lydia was my first close friend to get pregnant, and I knew it would mean a lot to her. I spent the afternoon enjoying the pink champagne and joking that all the oohing and aahing over the dinky baby outfits was perfect to satisfy any broody urges we might have lurking. To say babies were not on my radar would have been something of an understatement.

The next day I discovered I was pregnant. My first inkling that something was awry was in the car on the way to my sister's for Sunday lunch. We were definitely in a car, but hmmm, my stomach was churning as though I was on a boat in a storm. My brain began to race. Surely I hadn't had enough champagne yesterday for a hangover, had I? I never feel sick. This is not normal . . . When did I last have a period?

Will suggested that we stop and pick up a pregnancy test kit but I wasn't ready to cope with what it might say, so I said not to bother and tried to put the whole thing out of my mind. But I ended up dashing into Boots just before it shut that evening.

I'd love to say that Will and I cried with joy when we saw the little blue line, but the reality was that we hugged each other and prayed, shaking with nerves and adrenaline. I was grateful to God, but this was blended with a large dose of disbelief that I had got pregnant so quickly. I was in shock. I did another test immediately because I couldn't quite believe it was true.

Only six weeks previously we had stopped using contraception, perhaps naively assuming it would be a couple of years before I got pregnant. During the previous few years that Will had worked as a vicar, we had spent time with several couples facing the pain that comes with struggling to conceive. Subconsciously I expected that we too would travel down that road.

For the first few weeks of pregnancy I was in denial. I told my news to family and close friends, but felt disconnected from it, as though I was talking about something that was happening to someone else. I felt inadequate because I didn't feel broody and I found myself wondering what on earth you do with a baby. How do you even hold one?

The onset of full-on morning sickness was a helpful reminder that, while I might not feel ready for it, I really was carrying a life inside me and I had better start making adjustments accordingly.

## Your moment of discovery

I'd love to be a fly on the wall, watching those moments around the world when women discover they are pregnant and tell their partners. A whole variety of scenes must ensue – but perhaps the stereotypical image of this moment as conjured up during dreamy teenage years makes us expect that it should be one of sheer delight. However, the reality of life can mean that the beginning of the parenting journey may not be the idealized scenario we once expected. Author Elizabeth Martyn says, 'Becoming pregnant is the start of becoming a parent and marks the beginning of a long series of changes. Nothing is the same again from the moment you know you are pregnant.'[1] When you consider the life-altering potential of becoming pregnant, it is hardly surprising that our reaction to this news often encompasses a whole range of emotions.

Whatever your experience of the moment of discovering you were pregnant, God was there with you, and with the little life inside your body. An unborn life is infinitely precious to God, as Psalm 139 tells us. This psalm is unequivocal in its message that, while it may not feel like it at times, God has been in control of your life since your very first breath. As you look ahead, be reminded that he has plans to accompany you, and at times carry you, right through pregnancy.

Oh yes, you shaped me first inside, then out;
    you formed me in my mother's womb.
I thank you, High God – you're breathtaking!
    Body and soul, I am marvelously made!
    I worship in adoration – what a creation!
You know me inside and out,
    you know every bone in my body;
You know exactly how I was made, bit by bit,
    how I was sculpted from nothing into something.
Like an open book, you watched me grow from conception to birth;
    all the stages of my life were spread out before you,

The days of my life all prepared
   before I'd even lived one day.
(Psalm 139:13–16, *The Message*)

**How did you react when you first found out you were pregnant?**

'My mind was a whirl of thoughts. Firstly utter shock, then confusion, then excitement, then shock again . . . then amazement. I'm pleased to say that my husband was over the moon when I told him our news later that day, and now I am too.' Karen, thirty-six weeks pregnant

'My first thought was, "Brilliant! I've been waiting for this." It had taken me eighteen months to get pregnant. Sadly that pregnancy, which was with twins, ended in miscarriage. When I discovered I was pregnant the second time around, my reaction was very different. I was really, really worried.' Sam, mum to Charlie, three, and Jessica, one

'I was excited, scared and amazed all at once. I knew life was going to change from now on, which was scary, and I was worried about giving up my independence. I was quite aware of what hard work having children is, so I was also a little daunted.' Sarah, mum to Arthur, six months, and now twenty-two weeks pregnant

## The practical versus the spiritual

They say that in the final weeks before giving birth, pregnant women often get the urge to start spring-cleaning their houses. Balancing precariously on a chair while hoovering the top of your wardrobe with 8 lb of weight strapped to your tummy might sound like a ridiculously stupid thing to do, but trust me it does happen. As someone who normally detests cleaning, I secretly thought that pregnant women who had that 'problem' were a little strange. I told myself I'd never waste my time cleaning obsessively just before my baby came. But oh yes, to my total surprise, my hormonal clock kicked in at thirty-seven weeks to tell me it was time to prepare my home for the arrival of a new family member – and I don't think I've ever done so much housework in my life! I even rearranged all Will's theological books into thematic order, polished silver that hadn't seen a duster in five years and then hired a cleaner as a sort of bonus extra.

If you are nearing the end of your pregnancy, you may be well aware of the many things to consider in preparation for bringing a baby into your home. In the earlier months of pregnancy, there are other practical decisions to be made: Where will you have your baby? What sort of medical care do you want? Should you find out whether you are having a boy or a girl? Which hospital tests will you have? The lifestyle, dietary and exercise changes you need to make, and the impact of pregnancy on your work life, can all take over your thinking.

Somewhere inside, mum-to-be knows that preparing practically for baby is necessary, and many of these questions and issues do require careful thought. But sometimes it seems that an expectant mother will do – or buy – absolutely anything in a bid to give her new family member the best start in life. Don't make the mistake of squeezing God out of the picture by focusing solely on the practical preparations during this season of your life. I challenge you to ask him now to help you focus on him over and above the material, for the remainder of your pregnancy.

## God's view of pregnancy: three biblical birth stories

So what is God's view of pregnancy? If we are to look on this time through his eyes, what does he want us to see?

Throughout my pregnancy I devoured other women's birth stories, intrigued by what new mothers said about the build-up to 'B-day' and giving birth. (You'll find some birth stories with a difference in Chapter 6.) In the rest of this chapter I'm going to look at the birth stories of three women from the Bible who have inspired me: Eve, Elizabeth and Mary. You may already be very familiar with these stories, but reconsider them from your new perspective as a parent-to-be and you will be surprised at how you see them in a new light. Here, I hope to use them to map out God's view of pregnancy.

One difference you'll notice between the Bible's birth stories and those you read in magazines is the lack of gory detail in the biblical narratives. Luke's record of Mary giving birth to Jesus is one of very few biblical accounts of childbirth, and his mention of Elizabeth's baby John leaping 'for joy' in her womb (Luke 1:44) is one of only two times we read about a developing baby's activity during pregnancy.[2] Perhaps this is largely explained by the masculine authorship of the Bible – its writers had no first-hand experience of being pregnant. And first-century husbands would not normally have attended a child's birth, unlike many men today.

### *Eve: recognizes God's sovereign power*

Eve is the first pregnant woman mentioned in the Bible. She and Adam, as the first two humans that God has created, take up the command that God has given them to 'be fruitful and increase in number' (Genesis 1:28), and they have a child: 'Adam lay with his wife Eve, and she became pregnant and gave birth to Cain. She said, "With the help of the LORD I have brought forth a man." Later she gave birth to his brother Abel' (Genesis 4:1–2).

Eve's awareness that it is only with God's help that she is able to conceive and have children contrasts with our Western notion that having a child can be conveniently slotted into our life plans. I was hit by the reality of this philosophy through a series of TV documentaries that traced the stories of four women, all desperate to conceive, who were having difficulty in doing so. (I got totally hooked on the series during the early months of my pregnancy. Usefully, it coincided with the morning sickness days, many hours of which I spent lying on the sofa, feeling sorry for myself!) As their heart-wrenching stories unravelled, I was challenged: why was I not more grateful to God for conceiving without complications?

One woman was in her late thirties, single, and desperate to be a mother. This looked impossible from a natural perspective, and she was keen to adopt. She seemed ideal as an adoptive parent, but the process was slow and turbulent. She faced a series of painful disappointments as adoptions didn't work out at the last minute. Another single woman had IVF treatment, with a friend donating his sperm. He was uninterested in being the child's father, but simply wanted to do her a favour by enabling her to get pregnant.

While feeling compassion for these women who were bravely exposing their struggles on film – and resonating with their experiences in a new way because of my own sense of impending motherhood – the series also left me with deep-seated questions. Has having a child become little more than a woman's right?

So I had just got pregnant, and having been a Christian since the age of eleven, I knew God was Creator of all things, but was I giving him due recognition for his involvement as Eve had done? In a culture where we can choose our contraceptive methods, it's easy to forget that our ability to procreate comes through and from God alone. In having a child, Will and I were reflecting the creativity intrinsic to God's nature – and living out our calling to be in God's image in a whole new way. It is no mistake that the first mention of human procreation in Genesis 4 comes only two chapters after the description of God's resplendent act of creating the world in Genesis 1 and 2.

In God's eyes, a child is a gift given by him, whether we conceive naturally or with the help of IVF.[3] American author Elizabeth A. Hambrick-Stowe puts it like this:

> Pregnancy, the carrying of children, touches so intimately the
> original pattern of God in evoking new life that it expresses
> our human ability and opportunity with special power. This
> resonance with the divine is, in fact, the source of conception and
> pregnancy's excitement and desirability. Even people with no
> religious faith may sense something of this . . .[4]

Eve's birth story lay down a challenge for me: would I give God the glory for his gift, his work and this amazing opportunity?

While reflecting on the Bible's first mother, let's give a thought to her experience of giving birth. We find out about this in Genesis 3. After learning that Adam and Eve have disobeyed God by eating fruit from the forbidden tree, God tells them of the repercussions of their sinfulness. Genesis 3:16 says:

> To the woman he said,
>     'I will greatly increase your pains in childbearing;
>         with pain you will give birth to children.

> Your desire will be for your husband,
>> and he will rule over you.'

This is one biblical verse that has always upset me. Man seems to get off pretty lightly when it comes to repercussion for sin – his punishment is to have to toil the ground for the rest of his days in order to eat. But as far as I can tell, women have always toiled (and I expect forever will) just as hard as men, and we get pain in childbirth thrown in too! Why would God decide to make something as beautiful as bringing a baby into the world a thing of discomfort and pain?

As we think about this tricky little verse, we need to hold on to the truth that, as followers of Jesus, we are forgiven for our wrongs and restored to right relationship with him. The pain we experience in childbirth is therefore no longer a punishment for sin: Jesus took that punishment on himself on the cross. However, just as the reality is that men must still toil, so the legacy of a fallen human race is that women must struggle in labour. 'Labour' literally means hard work, and clearly nothing has changed in that department since the beginning of time!

The apostle Paul underlines this when he uses childbirth as a metaphor for explaining the suffering in the world, and how this suffering will exist until the kingdom of God comes fully when Christ returns. In Romans 8:22–23 we read,

> We know that the whole creation has been groaning as in the pains of childbirth right up to the present time. Not only so, but we ourselves, who have the firstfruits of the Spirit, groan inwardly as we wait eagerly for our adoption as sons, the redemption of our bodies.

So for Paul, birthing pain is a reminder that we are still part of the 'now' as well as the 'not yet' of the kingdom of God.

### Elizabeth: the miracle conception

Our second birth story comes in the first chapter of Luke's Gospel. Mary's cousin Elizabeth miraculously falls pregnant. She and her husband Zechariah were 'well on in years', and they were convinced that she would never have children.

The story reminds us of when Abraham and Sarah, in Genesis 17, are told by God that, although they are ninety-nine and ninety respectively, they will have a son. They name him Isaac (which means 'he laughs') as an expression of their happiness at having an unexpected child. Likewise in the first chapter of 1 Samuel, Hannah (whose womb, we are told, was closed) miraculously conceives and gives birth. She has cried out to God in prayer for a child and she calls her son Samuel, which means 'heard of God', 'because I asked the LORD for him' (1 Samuel 1:20).

With around one in seven couples in the UK struggling to conceive, Elizabeth's birth story, like Sarah's and Hannah's, offers hope for those facing this difficult issue. God really can, when he chooses, create life where physiology or medicine might have dictated this as being impossible.

One of the most amazing aspects of pregnancy for me was finally allowing my body to be the creative force it was designed to be. I marvelled at how it instinctively knew what to do at each stage through my pregnancy. How much more amazing must this feel for someone who thought their body could not do what nature intended? When Elizabeth finds out she is not barren as she had thought, but has in fact conceived, she rushes in to acknowledge the intervention of God in her life, just as Eve had done. Bubbling over with surprise, joy and excitement, she says, 'The Lord has done this for me' (Luke 1:25).

Elizabeth's pregnancy is deeply significant in kingdom terms, partly because it foretells her cousin Mary's. The child

Elizabeth is carrying grows up to become John 'the Baptist', who prepares the way for Jesus and had the privilege of baptizing him. However, feminist thinking has left us with the perception that having a child can mean the end (or at least a big disruption) to a woman's career, her independence and even her significance in the world. Naomi Stadlen, psychotherapist and mother of three, writes,

> Mothers can now take 'maternity leave' or plan a 'career break', but the assumption is that this is a short-term arrangement. Babies are regarded as an interruption to the normal flow of work. This can encourage a mother to see her employment as more important than having a baby. Mothers often report the shock of discovering that, after childbirth, their values reverse. For the first time, their employment, which meant a great deal to them before, can look less important than the baby.[5]

While becoming a parent does mean becoming less selfish, reassessing your priorities and making some life changes, Elizabeth's story is a reminder that motherhood in itself can be an incredibly exciting open door into the next stage of God's plan for your life. The shifts you need to make are worth it because of what God has in store for you as a parent. God will also have amazing kingdom plans and purposes for your child, just as he did for Elizabeth's son, John. Jeremiah 29:11 tells us, '"For I know the plans I have for you," declares the LORD, "plans to prosper you and not to harm you, plans to give you hope and a future."'

### Mary: the ultimate birth story ever recorded
One of the funniest twists in the tale of my pregnancy was that my baby's due date was 25 December. With Will being a vicar, we never heard the end of the jokes about

live-link-to-hospital nativity plays and whether we would name the baby Jesus, Holly or Noel.

My maternity leave spanned December, and during that time I delved back into Mary's birth story, recorded in the early chapters of Matthew's and Luke's Gospels. While I felt I knew the stories of the annunciation (Mary being told by the angel Gabriel that she is pregnant) and the incarnation (Jesus being born to a virgin mother) like the back of my hand, I found that, during this time, these narratives fascinated me as never before.

Mary's pregnancy obviously differs a little from yours or mine – she had the terrifying privilege of carrying the Son of God in her womb! She must have been torn between utter disbelief and alarm as the angel told her, 'The Holy Spirit will come upon you, and the power of the Most High will overshadow you. So the holy one to be born will be called the Son of God' (Luke 1:35).

The story of this incredible moment of discovery reminds us once again of the power of God to enable even the most miraculous of conceptions. Mary is told twice she has 'found favour' with God and so has been chosen to take part in his plans through her motherhood (Luke 1:28, 30). While your pregnancy and mine might feel as though they have nothing of the significance of Mary's, we too are part of the miracle that is conception, childbirth and motherhood. We are also specially favoured in our simply being able to have a child. In a sense, each pregnancy God gives is a reflection of that ultimately significant pregnancy, which brought his Son into our world.

Having gone to share her incredible news with her cousin Elizabeth, Mary sings a song of joyful praise to God for the pregnancy he has given her. This is known as Mary's song. It begins:

My soul glorifies the Lord
   and my spirit rejoices in God my Saviour,
for he has been mindful
   of the humble state of his servant.
From now on all generations will call me blessed,
   for the Mighty One has done great things for me –
   holy is his name.
(Luke 1:46–49)

The characters who play a part in the continuation of Mary's birth story also express the wonder and worship she shows in that spontaneous song of praise. Shepherds, angels and wise men worship at the sight of her newborn Son and glorify him as God.

Mary's attitude from the time she is told she will give birth to the Son of God, through to becoming a parent, challenged me profoundly. Her outlook displays little of the flurry of anxiety, stress and activity that I found myself falling into as I tried to prepare for giving birth while juggling other demands.

This is even more miraculous when you think about how becoming pregnant as an unmarried virgin would have been received in her culture: not very well! When the angel tells Mary that she will become pregnant, she is engaged to Joseph, but as they are not yet married, she has to deal with this news alone. Mary must have experienced the sort of isolating fear that only those parenting alone must know. She has no husband or partner to lean on – this moment is simply about her and God.

Mary must also have wondered whether her impending marriage would now even happen – surely Joseph would be suspicious of her 'an-angel-told-me-I-am-going-to-become-miraculously-pregnant' story? For Mary, rejection by family, friends and society at large was a real prospect. Death by stoning – the punishment due an adulteress – could await her, unless Joseph had the faith to believe her incredible story of God's intervention in her life, and to protect and support her in her new mission.

This makes it all the more amazing that after the annunciation, Mary's simple response to the news is to accept God's will, saying: 'I am the Lord's servant' (Luke 1:38). She goes on to endure a nightmare journey to Bethlehem, probably on the back of a donkey while heavily pregnant (that puts my complaints about no seat on the Tube to shame), and faces the impracticalities of giving birth in a smelly stable. Despite this, she is seemingly uncomplaining and somehow manages to rely on God, as her Son's birth takes place in the way the angel foretold.

Emphasizing that the strange events surrounding Jesus' birth really were a part of God's plan, Luke tells us that its timing was perfect. He writes: '. . . the time came for the baby to be born' (Luke 2:6). As I neared my impractical Christmas due date, I held on to this verse as a reminder that God knew just when my child would be born. He can bring on a birth at the ideal moment for the health of mother and baby. And with this little verse Luke also makes an important point about God's timing in sending his Son into the world – Jesus was born at just the right time to bring salvation to a desperate human race.

Mary manages to be deeply reflective about all God is doing in her life as she enters the new season of parenthood. She 'treasured up' all the unusual goings-on surrounding Jesus' birth, pondering on them in her heart (Luke 2:19). In an era when childbirth was without pain relief and brought with it the possibility of death – and having had a pretty

turbulent experience of early motherhood too – Mary is the
epitome of a trusting, faith-filled mother.

As you journey the unknown road of a first pregnancy,
Eve, Elizabeth and Mary are figures to look to for inspiration. They remind me that this time of my life can be done
God's way. When the pregnancy road is a rocky one, let's
remember Mary and her uncomfortable donkey trek to
the humble destination of her Son's birth. We really can
resonate with her, knowing that the mother of God faced
the grittiest of human circumstances as she brought her Son
into the world.

## For reflection or discussion

1. How did you react to the news that you were /
   your spouse was pregnant? Were the emotions you
   experienced different from what you expected?
2. If you were to estimate how much time you are
   spending preparing practically for having a baby, versus
   time spent prayerfully reflecting or talking with your
   spouse about the changes ahead, what would the ratio
   be? How can you change this?
3. Reread Mary's birth story in Luke 1 – 2. What is God
   teaching you through her journey to becoming a
   parent?

## 2. FROM LAD TO DAD: PREPARING FOR FATHERHOOD

**By Will**

I had always imagined I would be over the moon when I found out my wife was expecting our first baby. Instead, all I could muster was a weak 'Really?'

Of course all thse bravado would come later. I had a fresh sense of my own masculinity: I was a dad! But I was also aware that whilst many men have functional sperm, not every man makes a great parent. As Kent Nerburn said in *Letters to My Son*, 'It is much easier to become a father than to be one.'[1]

I have always been open to having children, and indeed my friends predicted I would be the first to be a father. But much as I might have worried my parents during my rebellious student years, no love children ever made an appearance! Instead I eventually found deep faith in Jesus. I don't know why, but I had always imagined marrying someone older, perhaps someone with a chequered relational history. Instead God blessed me with a wife who was younger and infinitely more beautiful than expected.

So, far from needing to heed a ticking biological clock, investing in marriage time was the order of the day. For five years life was a two-player game. The friends who had anticipated I would be the first father in our group now had two- and three-year-olds. They were probably starting to wonder if I had stood for too long in front of the microwave.

Having children with Louie was always there somewhere in the back of my mind, but sex had transitioned away from its procreative function, and for me it was with a level of disengagement that previously routine precautions were left in the drawer. Was fatherhood meant to be so unconsidered? Should I have prayed for the right time, or sought the Lord for his favour? I did neither – I merely enjoyed the moment.

Oh dear, my congregation aren't going to like this. I sound so trivial, so unspiritual. Surely as a vicar there must have been some deep, biblical wisdom I had meditated upon before trying for a child? Well, maybe I would have, if things hadn't happened so quickly. Don't we always get spiritual when things aren't going our way? Instead of undergoing preparative lament, I found myself in shocked thanksgiving: 'Dear Lord, thank you so much for Louie being pregnant. Sorry I didn't talk it all through with you earlier. I know you're in charge, and that's good, because I'm definitely not.'

## A new set of concerns

In my experience, something weird happens when the line goes blue. Two independent adults, bonded by love and marriage, become two needy and frightened oversized children bonded by love, marriage and a microscopic collection of quickly multiplying cells. Suddenly your self-interested fears: 'Am I going to get a promotion? Does my car tax need renewing? Shall I go running today?' are replaced by completely alien concerns, concerns that you didn't even know you should be concerned about: 'Shouldn't you be sitting down, darling? Are you sure you can still go to the shops? Have you had any of those follicle – or is it folic – acid pills today?'

### Joseph: dad-to-be in shock

Some people have even bigger early fears about becoming a parent. Take Mary's fiancé Joseph – a simple, first-century carpenter – for example. Here is a guy who is happily enjoying his engagement when it transpires his virginal bride-to-be is with child. Fortunately, to make things simpler, an angel appears in his dream to let him know that Mary hasn't cheated on him, but that she is pregnant with God's Son! You can imagine him wondering one minute: 'Did I oil my lathe today? Did I lock my workshop? Maybe I will try my hand at an ornate table leg tomorrow.' And the next: 'I wonder if God's Son has any special dietary requirements? What about that census in Bethlehem? Can I call myself the godfather or am I just a bystander?'

Joseph's initial plan on hearing that Mary was pregnant was to divorce her quietly, as he didn't want to expose her to the public disgrace of being pregnant outside of wedlock (Matthew 1:19). However, the angel he saw in his dream told him:

> Joseph son of David, do not be afraid to take Mary home as your
> wife, because what is conceived in her is from the Holy Spirit.
> She will give birth to a son, and you are to give him the name
> Jesus, because he will save his people from their sins.
> (Matthew 1:20–21)

Having obeyed the angel's words and married Mary (Matthew 1:24), Joseph then dealt with the situation in a practical, down-to-earth way. He fulfilled the legalities of a Roman census, making the necessary arrangements for a pregnant woman to go on a long journey. Although we might be critical of Joseph's booking of hostelries, he certainly was resourceful in the face of a crisis (Luke 2:1–7).

Sometimes I wonder what was going on in Joseph's heart through the nine months of Mary's pregnancy, knowing that his wife was carrying the Son of God. Peter J. Mead explores this in his poem, 'The Heart of the Matter':

> Could Joseph,
> a man accustomed to the rhythms of the workshop,
> of beating hammer and strumming saw,
> lean low and,
> placing his ear
> upon Mary's swollen belly,
> hear
> ('whoosh, whoosh, whoosh, whoosh')
> the parade of promises marching to be met
> ('whoosh, whoosh, whoosh, whoosh')
> the tyrannical empires of darkness toppling
> ('whoosh, whoosh, whoosh, whoosh')
> the stranglehold of sin released
> ('whoosh, whoosh, whoosh, whoosh')
> the beating heart of the living God?
>
> What else could account for his awed silence?[2]

## Responding to the big news

How you respond in the early stages of your wife's pregnancy may appear instinctive. However, it is more likely to be a blend of your own upbringing, values and desires. Rather than riding the wave of this heady concoction, it may help to be a bit more intentional. Ask yourself: 'What is my default response to the news that I will soon be a father?' But don't leave it there, pray into your answer to this question, and change things according to what God impresses upon you.

I'm going to take a closer look at some common masculine responses to pregnancy . . .

### DIY Dave

Some men naturally shift into DIY mode. Dave busies himself with all manner of practical concerns, trawling the Internet for a bargain Bugaboo pram, building his own MDF changing table and a bespoke baby-intercom unit.

It is perfectly natural to want to be a participant in pregnancy, and as your biological contribution has already been made, practical jobs can be a good outlet. However, be aware of what feelings might be driving the need to 'have it all sorted'. Sometimes we launch forth with tasks that are attainable because we wish to avoid deeper feelings, perhaps feelings of fear and insecurity.

The reality of the magnitude of becoming a father cannot be summed up by the contents of your Mothercare trolley. We need to let go of our coping strategies and ask ourselves, 'How do I really feel about being a dad?' You may go on to complete your odour-free nappy bin, but in the process try to recognize and pray through some of the emotional challenges that you would otherwise have left unaddressed.

### Kelvin: the provider

Kelvin is a busy man, too busy in fact really to get all that involved in the early stages of pregnancy. Kelvin has it in his mind to 'provide' for his child, just as his father provided for his mother and their children. He feels the urge to condense the impact of childrearing into the most convenient moment between the closing of the Footsie 100 and the opening of the Dow Jones. It's not that Kelvin doesn't want to be more demonstrative; it's just that with all those hormones swirling about, someone has to be strong and keep the show on the road.

If your wife has just taken this section of the book and shoved it under your eye line asking: 'Does this remind you of anyone?!', just say 'Yes, Gordon Gekko, in the film *Wall Street* . . . but I'm nothing like him!' Kelvin's intentions are honourable, however, although I think he needs to think beyond the pregnancy and the birth to the lifelong journey of fatherhood. The reality is that life cannot be squeezed into convenient moments, and finances are not everything. God has called you to fatherhood, and that encompasses so much more than practical provision for your family. Investing yourself emotionally now will help you to calibrate to the changes that fatherhood brings. While providing for your family is significant, nothing can be a substitute for the silent or verbal expression of your love, both for your spouse and your child.

### Over-eager Simon

Over-eager Simon is a fountain of knowledge. He has already consumed the whole of *The Contented Little Baby Book* by Gina Ford and, in the spirit of his university debating society, he takes the opportunity to argue the case for scheduled feeding over the 'evils' of routine-free parenting. Simon's wife has neither the energy nor the inclination to enter into a neonatal version of *The Krypton Factor* and so he is relegated to pitting himself against the wits of his unmarried mates at The Red Lion on a Friday night. This, as you can imagine, does little to harness the imagination or goodwill of those not yet in the baby way.

One can't help but notice a deep insecurity in the way Simon is approaching fatherhood. In a similar way to both Dave and Kelvin, he longs to keep the boundaries of parenting clear, and he is trying to pass the test for knowledge, as if understanding everything will make it all go well. Sadly, useful as some knowledge is, in the process of attaining it he is withdrawing real support from his spouse, and alienating valuable friends.

By virtue of the fact that you are reading this book, it's likely that you are aware of the vast quantity of knowledge that surrounds pregnancy and parenting. And I am sure it is not unjustified to say that some marketing plays upon the fears and insecurities of parents-to-be. The must-knows, must-dos and must-haves can all become a pressurized holy grail for the well-intentioned parent, sadly to the detriment of valuable emotional and spiritual calibration for parenthood. But the premise of this book is that pregnancy is an utterly unique and God-given opportunity to prepare yourself for the changes ahead as you reach fatherhood. In the life of your child, this is the only period of preparation you will have. From the moment of birth you are living fatherhood, reacting, adapting, and wishing you had prepared more!

### Zechariah: disbelieving dad-to-be

At the beginning of Luke's Gospel we find two deeply contrasting stories of preparation for parenthood. Louie has already explored Mary's response to the news that she would become a parent (in Chapter 1), and here I am going to look at the very different story of Zechariah receiving the news that he will be a father in his old age.

In Luke 1:8–9 we see that Zechariah, a priest, was chosen to go into the Holy of Holies to renew the incense to be burned before the Lord. Lots were drawn over which priest would perform this terrifying role. A rope was tied around the priest's waist so that if he were to die in the Holy of Holies, his body could be pulled out and he would not defile the temple.

As you can imagine, Zechariah's preparations for this encounter with God behind the curtain were all-encompassing. However, on this particular journey into the temple, he is in for a shock. Zechariah comes face to face with the angel Gabriel, who says,

> Do not be afraid, Zechariah; your prayer has been heard. Your wife Elizabeth will bear you a son, and you are to give him the name John. He will be a joy and delight to you, and many will rejoice because of his birth, for he will be great in the sight of the Lord . . . he will be filled with the Holy Spirit even from birth. (Luke 1:13–15)

Sure beats a blue-line pregnancy test any day!

Oddly, rather than bowing and scraping in response, Zechariah questions the angel's news. In verse 18 he says, 'How can I be sure of this? I am an old man and my wife is well on in years.' Isn't this ironic? Here we have an old and eminently respected priest, going into the temple to perform a role that was deemed life-threatening because it might involve a face-to-face encounter with God. Yet when God's angelic envoy appears and tells him that he is going to be a father, he refuses to believe it. I wonder whether your reaction to the pregnancy test was one of disbelief?

Zechariah had all of the outward attributes of a well-respected priest and was practically prepared for what God might have for him, but his heart was not prepared at all.

God strikes Zechariah silent because of his faithless response to the news that he will soon be a father. The angel Gabriel also instructs Zechariah to call his son John, which means in Hebrew, 'The Lord is gracious.' In verse 61 we see that his relatives think this is an odd idea, since no-one in their family has that name. This is the key point here: Zechariah feels shame at the absence of a descendant and he disbelieves Gabriel because he knows it is physically impossible for Elizabeth to bear a child. So when it comes to naming his son, he has a significant choice to make. Either he can remain proud and name his son after himself, or he can humble himself and attribute the child appropriately to God's hand. Because Zechariah has been struck dumb, he asks for a writing tablet, and on it he puts, 'His name is John' (Luke 1:63). The couple's neighbours and relatives are astonished, and they must have been even more surprised when on making this decision, Zechariah is suddenly once again able to speak.

By naming his baby John, Zechariah was forgoing the honour that was given to a father in the first century. He was handing over his pride and releasing the child to the ownership of the Lord.

Zechariah's story is a messy one, but it does end well. It contains some really painful issues: the struggle through infertility, disbelief at pregnancy, family interference, and releasing a child to God. You may resonate with just one or many of these issues, but however you feel, this story brings comfort, reminding us that we all face challenges in calibrating to fatherhood. The great news is that we also have the chance to lay down an incredible legacy for our children.

Zechariah may have struggled to accept that he would be a father in the first instance, but he obviously did a fantastic job of fathering his son. John the Baptist was a picture of integrity and holiness. Gordon MacDonald writes:

If there is one thing that begins to explain John, it has to be
the kind of parents he had, who shaped him in his earliest days
. . . We have little indication of John's family life after he was
born, but we do know that his parents were marked with an
extraordinary depth of integrity, godliness and perseverance.[3]

## Preparing to be out of control

Zechariah was an older man whose life pattern was probably
fixed before fatherhood. Hearing the news that he was going
to become a dad was a huge shock, but one he would ultimately adapt to. Becoming a parent will change things, but
rather than think about how to limit the changes, why not
reflect on how you feel about not being in control? Much of
our ability to become competent fathers will depend upon
our ability to embrace change.

When Louie was pregnant, nothing irritated me more
than other dads raising their eyebrows and saying, 'Of
course, life will never be the same', or 'Get ready for a life
catastrophe!' They made me feel angry and competitive. I
would think, 'Don't project your incompetence on to me,
just because you can't handle having a baby!'

My aggressive reaction was part of my defence system.
I was assuring myself that I wouldn't let things change.
But the trouble with my mentality was that it is reductive:
'I'm holding on tightly until I'm forced to do otherwise!'
Had I carried on thinking like this, life could have become a
desperate wrestle between previous priorities and the new
demands that fatherhood brings.

Not every man has a competitive attitude, but many of us
have been trained to find a competition around every corner.
Competition in parenting is futile, however. This is firstly
because every child is different. Your own child's unique
needs and personality are the greatest influence on how you

raise him or her, regardless of how 'good' you think you are. The second reason to walk off the court is that your child will ultimately be the loser if you attempt to be 'super in control'. Whatever other dads tell you about their lifestyle, parenting or relationships, your experience will be different. A competition has rules, boundaries and equality – but your child needs flexibility and comprehension, not comparisons and unrealistic expectations.

The other loser in your attempt to mitigate the impact of fatherhood is your wife. During the first few months of becoming a mother she will need extra support and attention from you at times of day and night that simply can't be predicted. She may struggle with post-natal depression, which she can't explain or even readily acknowledge. She will certainly need extra help during her post-birth recovery, particularly if she has had a Caesarean.

In order to explore this further, try writing down your current life shape. You could do a pie chart or a doodle. What proportion of your time is spent working, relaxing, doing sport, extra activities and so on? Once you have a visual representation of your life's shape, it becomes easier to see what sort of challenges the demands of fatherhood are going to bring. Think about where on your pie chart you might create space for your new family member.

## Building in margin

One of my friends, Jonny, was given a Blackberry by his employer. He told me that, within a few weeks of having it in his possession, he found himself sitting on the toilet answering e-mails. He thought about it afterwards and said to me, 'I have got to hand it back . . . I can't even go to the loo in peace!' Jonny's experience is not unique. We live in a margin-free world where every moment is allocated. We don't need to wait for anything, and we have to schedule our time off, otherwise we just wouldn't get any. How is your child going to fit in to your margin-free world?

Before Louie gave birth, I thought how generous and prepared I was by allocating clear 'fathering' slots in my busy schedule (and packed pie chart). I was determined not to try to squeeze my child into my 'spare time', mainly because I don't know what 'spare' is! This might seem very well intentioned to you now, but it was in fact a mechanical view of fatherhood. I was saying, 'I'm going to pop you into my schedule.'

Note to self: in the early days, a baby doesn't do routine. Skye sometimes feeds for forty-five minutes, job done. Then she pukes up every last ounce of her milk and wants to start again. It isn't her fault; it is just something they call 'colic', and, believe me, Mr Colic is not your friend. The fact is, Skye needs my flexible, focused attention on demand. She has to drive it (within reason) according to the rhythms of her developing body and my loving wife's generosity. My life needs margin more than it needs a schedule. I need to allocate time for fatherly duties, but I also need to build more margin into my life so that Skye and I can be together as and when she most needs me.

There are two other important reasons why life margin is important for fatherhood.

## 1. Margin for you

Parenting is really tiring, even for the most energetic father. I expected that the first week would be shattering, but thought that I would soon find myself on the trajectory to recovery. The first four days were as expected, exhausting but also driven by an adrenaline high. However, over the next five weeks I felt progressively more tired. Fatherhood is as unrelenting as it is wonderful, and any margin I had previously built into my life for me had suddenly been swallowed up.

The reality of life without margin is a grumpy and semi-functional dad. Fatherhood can only really be enjoyed if you keep some time for a break. Look back at your life-shape picture and identify the things that refresh you. Now decide which of these you are going to build into your life as a father, and commit to maintaining them. I have always found that physical exercise gives me a good release and helps me to stay fresh, but in the past this has come in the shape of serious rowing which has taken up hours each week. I have learnt that team sports actually add a heavy pressure to my life and an obligation to team mates that I can no longer fulfil.

With this in mind, I have made exercise work for me by building it into my margin. Since having Skye, my gym trips have become difficult to manage during the early evening. Instead I have brought the gym to me with a couple of cheeky eBay purchases. Now I am saving money as well as fitting exercise in between Skye's bath time and our supper-time. I can even turn down the beans from my cross trainer!

The point of my sharing this small detail of my life is to encourage you that you can still do the things that restore you, but you may have to be more creative about the way you set them up. Remember that babies need regular atten-tion in short bursts. In the first months of fatherhood you may need to think about fitting activity or rest into slots of around forty-five minutes rather than three hours.

## 2. Margin for the sake of your marriage
You will also need margin for the benefit of you and your wife. Unless you are a stay-at-home dad, your fathering will look quite different from your spouse's mothering within the

first few months of your baby's life. This can cause tension and disputes at a time when your relationship is already under new pressure.

A shattered mother generally couldn't care less what you did at work today. In fact, your work, which used to be a source of sympathy, will become a luxury escape in her eyes. Therefore if you build no margin into your life and come home expecting to put your feet up, crack open a chilled bottle of beer and switch on the football, think again. It is of course really hard for dads who do go off to stressful jobs, only to come home to a new set of demands, but that is the reality you need to prepare yourself for.

If you build some down time into your working day, especially at lunch or as you travel home, you will be better able to release some pressure for your spouse when you get there. It is wise to get out of the mentality of expecting to rest in the first hour of getting home from work. Many mothers are desperate for a break by the time their husband returns. In the past, being half an hour late home would have meant nothing, but now being ten minutes late can cause major frustration for my clock-watching wife! Try hard to be back on time, and if you can't, regularly update her on your progress. If you come in with enthusiasm to take the baby or change a nappy, your relationship will really benefit.

There is no doubt that having a baby does affect your work – it is foolish to suppose otherwise. Be realistic and honest about what is happening at home. Your bosses are better off knowing and understanding why you seem tired or are unable to perform extra duties, rather than just thinking that you are reticent and unwilling. Many of them will be parents too and fully aware of what you are going through. Just one other thing to keep in mind: much as you try to regulate work, margin and home life, it won't always go to plan. Be patient with yourself and expect to take time to adjust things as you go along.

Building margin into your life is a practical activity. I know I am stating the obvious, but it is amazing how many of us will read about margin and agree wholeheartedly with the principle, yet do absolutely nothing about it. Having margin in your life is about actively choosing to create space; if you don't, it won't appear.

It is often when we take action that we begin to sense what is going on under the surface, what is holding us back and what we need to pray through. It is my hope that we will explore some of these hidden drivers later in the book. In the meantime, sit back with a nice cup of tea, and enjoy some margin in your life!

## Three practical ways to prepare for fatherhood

### 1. Get to know your unborn baby

There have been many scientific studies about the responsiveness of babies while still in the womb. These have shown that they respond to music, voices and even a touch on mummy's tummy. Bonding with your unborn baby can help you prepare for becoming a father, as you begin to build an emotional connection with your child. In *Best Things Fathers Do*, Will Glennon highlights the importance of establishing a connection with your baby before he or she is born:

> Fathers come to their children from the outside from the very beginning. We can participate in the progress of our wives' pregnancies, we can place our hands in strategic spots to feel the kicks and jabs . . . But our experience is always filtered; no matter how we participate, fundamentally we remain on the outside.
>
> In some profound way, our biological placement in the

process of birth mirrors the challenges we will face throughout our children's lives. For most mothers, the primary struggle of parenthood is stepping back far enough to allow the child the room to grow and develop. The challenge for most men, on the other hand, is coming in close enough so that we can build a strong and lasting bond.[4]

In the first instance, talking to your wife's bulging stomach can feel strange, if not a bit embarrassing. The thing is to persist and allow your self-consciousness gradually to disappear. Over the final few months of pregnancy, bonding with Louie's bump became great fun. I used gently to massage Bio Oil into her tummy, something which offered a number of different benefits, including protecting her skin from developing stretch marks, having a reason to spend an extended time facing her tummy, and doing something that helped us both to relax as parents. Chatting to our baby in the womb gradually crept into this routine as it became more natural. Nothing can really prepare you for the excitement of that little hand or foot first jabbing at you from under the skin.

As Christian parents, we also have the privilege of praying for our unborn baby. Try laying hands on mum's bump each night before going to sleep, and commit your child to Jesus.

## 2. Be informed

I have already stressed that knowledge is not everything in preparing for fatherhood. However, having a balanced and broad understanding of the basics of pregnancy and birth is really valuable. One of the best ways to do this, especially if the books send you to sleep, is to attend an NCT (National Childbirth Trust) course.[5] Both the NCT and your hospital will have practical sessions that prepare you for the birth and initial weeks with a newborn. Louie and I went on an intensive NCT weekend course which, despite my initial reluctance, turned out to be great fun. I realized that, by going, I was saying something important to Louie too. I was saying, 'We're in this together.' At one point I found myself changing the nappy of a particularly ugly Cabbage Patch doll in front of ten laughing dads-to-be. There was lots of nervous banter but also a real sense that we could actually be of some use when it came down to it.

### 3. Talk to other dads

Try asking some other dads what they love most about being a father. As I write this, five months into parenthood, I can genuinely tell you that being Skye's father is the most wonderful privilege I have ever had. At the end of a long day at work I rush home from my office, excited about seeing her smile and sharing a few giggles together as we do her bathtime routine. Have you let yourself think that you might actually really enjoy being a dad?

**What do you most enjoy about being a dad?**

'Seeing James change day by day, and watching him dance to the worship music in church.' Rob, dad to James, eight months

'A baby is the perfect reason to remove yourself from the centre of your own universe. It's great to think of someone else more that you think about yourself and your own life, struggles and triumphs. I enjoy understanding what so many of my friends and family have already been through.' Andrew, dad to Jack, eight weeks

'Seeing my children laugh. I love teaching them things, going on adventures with them and seeing how God has uniquely made each one.' Paul, dad to Sam, five, Owen, four and Hope, one

## For reflection or discussion

1. What sort of actions have you engaged in since discovering your wife was pregnant? What do these tell you about how you feel about becoming a father?
2. How might you build more margin into your life? In what ways might doing this affect your relationship with your wife and child?
3. Ask two friends what they love most about being dads.

## 3. FAITH OR FEAR? TRUSTING GOD THROUGH PREGNANCY

**By Louie**

'Will I miscarry before twelve weeks? Should I tell people I am pregnant when I could lose the baby after I've let them know? How will I deal with my body looking totally different? How would I react if our child was born with a serious illness?

'What will it be like to be a mum? Will I be bored out of my head? Will I love my baby when I finally see it for the first time – and if I don't, will I feel desperately guilty? How will my husband deal with becoming a dad? And how will I cope with the sleep deprivation?'

Pregnancy can do strange things to a woman. Even the most laid-back, level-headed character can find herself lost in a sea of worries when it comes to bringing a child into the world. Heather Best writes,

> Pregnancy is one of the most extreme times in a woman's
> life: extreme emotions, extreme moods, extreme appetite. I

remember being so tired, but also incredibly ambitious. I was nervous about the baby's health, doctor's visits, needles, and weight gain, and yet I understood real hope for the first time in my life.[1]

I met Sharon, a doctor, at antenatal NCT classes. She is possibly the friendliest, most relaxed and approachable doctor I've yet come across. Her baby was due three weeks before mine, and frustratingly for her, she went a week and a half overdue. At her forty-one-week hospital appointment to discuss possible induction, she had a wild diva fit (very out of character) and demanded that the consultant give her a Caesarean section then and there. As you can imagine, the consultant didn't oblige. Sharon was booked in for an induction a few days later, although to her relief, baby Kieran arrived naturally the day before the appointment. At some stage, every mother-to-be gets totally overwhelmed by the trials and concerns that pregnancy brings.

This was certainly true for me. Once I'd got used to the idea that I was actually going to have a baby, I found it hard not to worry throughout pregnancy. There were so many unknowns, more question marks than my head could handle. I mention a few of my fears and self-doubts above, and in this chapter I'll explore some of these in more detail.

In *The Best Friends' Guide to Pregnancy*, Vicki Iovine writes,

It is neck-snapping, the speed with which you can go from feeling joyous to feeling terrified upon learning that you are going to have a baby. First there is a sort of general sense of alarm at the whole prospect of growing a baby inside you and being responsible for it until the day you die. This is when you might start looking for an escape. Shortly after this, the fears become more specific.[2]

I wonder what specific fears are rattling around your head at the moment? For me, worry number one was whether the baby would be carried full term, and whether it would be healthy. When I went to see my GP for the first time after discovering I was pregnant, I was armed with a list of worried-sounding questions. She responded, 'Once the baby's born there will be far more to worry about – at least at the moment you can't see what's going on in there.'

Her pragmatic advice helped me realize that I had no real option: start praying and trust God, or stress out for the next nine months about all sorts of things I had no control over anyway. And the reality was that the stress-out option wouldn't be any good for the baby's development. I started asking God for strength to stop worrying and took practical steps to challenge my fears. Gradually fear began to lift. In its place started to come a deep assurance – a level of faith that I rarely find within myself – that, come what may, God was going to protect this baby.

## Worries, worries, worries

Despite knowing God's love and faithfulness, I still struggled not to worry about our baby's health as my pregnancy progressed. When I went to the doctor for my first prenatal appointment and she measured my bump to check the baby was growing healthily, we discovered that it was too small for the stage I was at. I was packed off to hospital that day for emergency checks and another scan.

This happened on one of the worst possible days – Will was hosting and speaking at the first Mind and Soul conference.[3] I decided not to call him about it until he'd finished his talk, as I knew his ability to focus would be ruined. I sat on the bus to the hospital, trying not to question everything, and clinging on to my faith that God had said he had this baby in his hands.

To our relief, the scan showed no problems with the baby. My bump was just on the small side of things. However, I had to have five extra, unexpected scans between then and the end of my pregnancy. Every time, I teetered on the edge of the pit of fear and had to force myself to grab on to God's goodness and promises lest I should slip in.

Pregnancy and birth processes are safer than ever before, something for which I am, of course, hugely thankful. But the extra knowledge we have (in comparison even to the previous generation) about how a pregnancy is developing can create so much more to worry about.

And it wasn't only medical factors that I worried about during pregnancy. Although Will and I had decided that we didn't want to find out the sex of our baby before birth, endless people took one glance at my bump and said it was definitely 'boy shaped'. Despite knowing that amateur 'bump shape analysis' is far from an advanced science, it was hard to ignore all those opinions. I ended up still trying to be open-minded, but deep down expecting to give birth to a boy. Then I began to worry about how I would feel if it was a girl after all. I felt bad that I was even bothered by this issue – shouldn't I just be delighted to have a healthy baby? As I explored these feelings, I started to realize that my fear was that if I had a daughter, she would be more likely to replicate my own issues and mistakes than a son would.

Trusting God through this meant coming back to the truth that he really can bring change, freedom and new life. By his power and through our constantly seeking to become more like him, there is no reason why our children – boys or girls – should struggle with the same things as their parents did. In retrospect, I am glad we didn't find out the sex of our child, because I feel it taught me early on to start trusting for the other total unknowns that parenthood would throw my way. I had to let go of my urge to plan and prepare everything. When I finally saw our baby – a girl – the surge of love I felt for her was overwhelming. I have realized that, son or daughter, God is faithful in equipping us to love our children as they need to be loved, and to delight in them whoever they turn out to be.

### What were your greatest fears during pregnancy?

'My biggest worry through pregnancy was the prospect of labour! I remember worrying on countless occasions that I might die during labour, but my family reassured me that the doctors and midwives deliver thousands of babies every year. My other concern was my age: at twenty-six, were we too young to start a family? It meant I didn't have a group of friends who I could turn to during this new phase of my life.' Lydia, mum to Harry, eighteen months

'I found the changes to my body shape hard to adjust to. My husband has always found me attractive during pregnancy, but as I put on a lot of weight and was very hormonal during my first pregnancy, I didn't feel attractive most of the time.' Sarah, mum to Arthur, six months, and now twenty-two weeks pregnant

'I worried about the health of the baby. You can see and hear how your wife is doing, but you don't have much to go on with the baby. When it came to the ultrasound, I couldn't wait to take a look at him – but when you see his body, your mind instantly fills with often unspoken questions: "Is it normal that his head or belly can really be that big? And his heartbeat – why is it so fast?" The kicking also worried me. It's great when it gets regular, but then it stops – sometimes for days – and you think, "Is he alright? What does it mean?"' Andrew, dad to Jack, eight weeks

## Your companion on the journey ahead: fear or faith?

Perhaps what stands out to me most about the birth stories of Eve, Elizabeth and Mary that we looked at in Chapter 1 is that fear does not appear to play a dominant part in any of their experiences. My suspicion, though, is that like every parent-to-be, these women were in fact worried and fearful at different stages during their pregnancies.

If fear has been your main companion during pregnancy so far, and you relate strongly to the questions and worries mentioned in this chapter, don't feel isolated. You are not alone. Think about how Mary must have felt: how could anybody find out they were going to be the mother of the Saviour of the world and not feel just a little bit edgy? What we can learn from her and these other biblical parents-to-be is that fear does not have to take over during this time in our lives. Despite their worries, Eve, Elizabeth and Mary managed to trust God and look to him as their source of strength.

For those who have a traumatic pregnancy, holding on to belief in God can be incredibly tough. Tracy goes to church with a friend of mine in Phoenix, USA. The story of her pregnancy with her daughter Anna gives substance to the truth that we really can have faith – and see God move miraculously – in the sort of circumstances that form the stuff of every parent-to-be's nightmare.

## Tracy's story

Tracy found out at fifteen weeks that her baby had a serious condition known as a diaphragmatic hernia.[4] Her doctors later told her that Anna also had severe heart problems, and their advice was to terminate the pregnancy.

'Listening to the doctors' disregard for my child's life left me ready to fight,' she says of her decision to go ahead with the pregnancy. She was to endure twenty-five further weeks of fraught concern and endless medical appointments. Her walk with God through this time was difficult. 'Part of me shut down. It was just too much to work with. So I kind of emotionally disconnected. On a head level, I knew I needed God to get me through this and I believed he answered prayer, but my own faith was shaky. I did believe in the power of other people's faith, so on a lot of days, asking others to pray was my prayer,' she says.

Tracy tells of how faithful God was during this traumatic season. 'After one particularly troubling doctor's appointment during which I was told that Anna's heart problem was getting worse, I came home and read the assigned Gospel text for the day – it was the story of Jesus healing the man's daughter, even though it seemed that she had died. In it Jesus says, "Don't be afraid; just believe" (Mark 5:36). It was one of those times when the words jump off the page and you absolutely know he is speaking to you. I held on to those words, especially during the last month of pregnancy.'

Tracy went to a prayer group on Sunday nights throughout her pregnancy. 'Those prayers on Sunday nights brought shifts (both in my spirits and in Anna's health) when nothing else seemed able to help,' she recalls. 'The fact that this group of people believed that God would break through the heavens to change the health of this child inside me was so powerful. These people were not just praying, "God's will be done" in this situation; they were praying "Your kingdom come, Lord. And let it break into our lives through the healing of this child."'

During Tracy's labour, friends came to the hospital and prayed in the chapel for her and the baby. 'Two hours after Anna was born, the doctors began murmuring that they could not find the hernia,' she says. 'A few days later they were willing to say it definitively: the condition that had been diagnosed by three different groups of doctors before Anna arrived was no longer there. The heart defect was now just a mild anomaly. Although Anna has a small left lung and a bad case of reflux, the surgeries and treatments we had been warned about were not necessary. None of the doctors even tried to give a medical explanation and one couple went as far as to use the word "miracle",' says Tracy.

Reflecting on her experience of pregnancy, she concludes, 'My understanding of healing is still evolving, but one of the most important things I learned from this experience is that my faith didn't heal Anna. The Lord did. I had no idea what he was going to do – and on some days last summer I really did believe the worst reports. Fear got the better of me more often than not. But God heard the cries of his saints, people from all over the world who were praying for Anna, and answered them.'

## What's pressing your worry buttons?

For many of us, particular past events – and even the experiences of our close friends or family members – can leave us with one or two particularly potent fears. Susanna, mum to eight-month-old James, felt that for much of her pregnancy a cloud of fear about losing her baby hung over her head. Susanna had previously miscarried, which made her terrified

that the same thing would happen again. But her fears were
also exacerbated by the tragic and extremely rare experience of a close friend, whose baby sadly died when she was
forty weeks pregnant. Although Susanna has always loved
the worship song 'I Surrender All' by Judson Van Deventer,
during her pregnancy she found herself almost unable to
say those words to God. Could she really trust him with the
child she had longed for? Susanna knew she needed to trust
that God was able to protect her own life and her child's,
but this was a very real struggle for her.

In her book *Good Enough Mother*, Naomi Starkey explores
the subject of the ambitions we have for our children – and
the disappointment our children may also cause us at different times in our lives.

> For most of us, the morning sickness stage has barely passed
> before the thoughts [about ambition] begin to take shape. How
> good-looking will my child be? How intelligent? How popular?
> While we may not get down to the specifics prenatally ('I'm
> going to give birth to a dark-haired six-foot rugby international,
> with a doctorate in economic theory'), how many of us have
> not started dreaming dreams as we watch our little one begin to
> explore the world?[5]

If we aren't worrying about the course our pregnancy is
taking and our developing baby's health, we may instead
be concerned about what his or her future might be – and
whether it will live up to our hopes. We may wonder: What
might God call my child to? Will I have it in me to love and
accept my son, whatever path he makes his own? What
will my daughter's future choices say about her parents?
There is an inevitability about pregnancy that terrified me
at times: I would need to parent not only a baby, but also a

toddler, a teenager and one day an adult. This was a lifelong responsibility!

Do you find a certain fear constantly cropping up during your – or your spouse's – pregnancy? Can you recognize cycles of worry that keep resurfacing?

## In whom are we trusting?

As we think again about the kind of God we are called to trust through pregnancy, I want to turn to the Old Testament use of parenting and birth imagery.

In the book of Isaiah, the prophet tells of how the people of Israel have been disobedient to God, and a chasm has developed between him and them. They suspect that God has abandoned them. Isaiah draws on childbirth imagery to express that this is not in God's nature. God is like a devoted mother who cannot desert the child she loves and has birthed:

> But now listen, O Jacob, my servant,
>     Israel, whom I have chosen.
> This is what the LORD says –
>     he who made you, who formed you in the womb,
>     and who will help you:
> Do not be afraid, O Jacob, my servant,
>     Jeshurun, whom I have chosen.
> (Isaiah 44:1–2)

These verses remind us that the God we struggle to trust through our pregnancies once watched over us in our own mother's womb. He doesn't overlook our prayers and pleas to him to be close to us and protect us and our unborn child. He is ready and willing to help us, and his message is not to be afraid, because he has not forgotten us.

Isaiah repeats this, using childbirth and parenting imagery once again, in chapter 49:

> But Zion said, 'The LORD has forsaken me,
>     the Lord has forgotten me.'
>
> 'Can a mother forget the baby at her breast
>     and have no compassion on the child she has borne?
> Though she may forget,
>     I will not forget you!'
> (Isaiah 49:14–15)

Later on in Isaiah we see that God promises to bring an end to the pain and distress of his estranged people. He will intervene in their situation, bringing good out of hardship. This is paralleled by the joy of actually having a child, after the pain of labour has been endured.

> 'Do I bring to the moment of birth
>     and not give delivery?' says the LORD.
> 'Do I close up the womb
>     when I bring to delivery?' says your God.
> (Isaiah 66:9)

Isaiah also reminds us in chapter 66 that God, again like a deeply caring mother, will comfort us through all we face. He brings us hope and restoration following times of worry and distress. God says:

> As a mother comforts her child,
>     so will I comfort you;
>     and you will be comforted over Jerusalem.
> (Isaiah 66:13)

## Jesus and the fear factor

In the Gospels, faith and fear are regularly juxtaposed – Jesus challenges his disciples to be people of faith instead of people of fear. The story of Jesus calming the storm encapsulates his message:

> One day Jesus said to his disciples, 'Let's go over to the other side of the lake.' So they got into a boat and set out. As they sailed, he fell asleep. A squall came down on the lake, so that the boat was being swamped, and they were in great danger.
>
> The disciples went and woke him, saying, 'Master, Master, we're going to drown!'
>
> He got up and rebuked the wind and the raging waters; the storm subsided, and all was calm. 'Where is your faith?' he asked his disciples.
>
> In fear and amazement they asked one another, 'Who is this? He commands even the winds and the water, and they obey him.'
> (Luke 8:22–25)

Your pregnancy may be like sailing on calm waters, or it may be that storms rage in your life during this time. I encourage you to invite Jesus into your boat wherever you are on this trip. Let him be your companion on this unique journey, not sitting beside you as you try to maintain the upper hand – but let him direct your ship.

## The power of prayer

Committing your unborn baby to God in prayer is the most powerful way to overcome the fears you face during pregnancy. Prayer can actually transform your child's life, both now and in his or her future. In *Praying for Your Unborn Child*, Francis and Judith MacNutt write:

We are convinced that extraordinary changes in the health and happiness of children will take place if you really believe that Jesus – that prayer – can make a real difference. Psychiatrists, such as Dr. Thomas Verny, are saying that the unborn child picks up on his parents' feelings and thoughts in an extraordinary way and that the greatest help or detriment in determining the child's emotional and physical health is the mother's attitude towards the fetus . . .

What more beautiful way of turning the love of mother and father toward that child than when they are praying together![6]

Have you just felt a pang of guilt that you haven't been praying for your child enough? I found myself asking, 'What if I have already damaged or disadvantaged my child by my flimsy prayer life?' Don't let your guilt that you haven't been praying stop you from starting. I read the MacNutts' little book on the Tube to and from work during pregnancy. I was inspired to pray for my baby more than I had been doing previously, and I started using my commute specifically as a time to pray for her.

Praying for the baby with Will also drew us together as we brought our worries and fears to God. This can also build a really healthy habit of prayer for your future family life. Cath, mum to Ridley, thirteen months, and Bethan, one week, said, 'Throughout pregnancy we committed to pray for our child, and for ourselves as a family – that God would protect us, prepare us and fill our baby with his Holy Spirit. This has continued as we try to spend time with our son and God each day. I think I have been struck most by the need for his guidance and wisdom. We all want to be the very best parents we can be, and I know I need help to be that.'

## Practical steps

Understanding the faithfulness of God in the face of fear, and bringing our concerns to him in prayer, are the most important things we can do when worry strikes. However, as well as this, there are a number of practical tools we can use to combat worry.

### 1. Get specific

Worries tend to be very general and often morph from one thing to another. But by being specific about your worries and bringing them into the light, they lose their power and become less frightening. Try writing down your top ten worries as a succinct list and pray through them every day. The more you look at them, the less frightening they will become. This is a tool called 'exposure response prevention'. Share the specifics of your worries and pray about them with your spouse or a trusted friend. If you are reading this as a husband whose wife is pregnant, have you encouraged her to do this?

### 2. Think about your physical condition

Your physical condition will have a great impact on the way that your mind receives potential threats. When you are over-tired, feeling low about yourself, hungry or unwell, you will almost always feel more anxious than normal. Try and journal when you feel most susceptible to worries during your day, and plan to pray, do an activity, or chat to a friend during that time the next day or week. Distraction can be a healthy technique to prevent worry from taking hold. Equally, if you find yourself consumed by a specific worry, choose to do something practical to break the cycle, like going for a brisk walk in the park.

### 3. Relaxation techniques

Our brains have a very sensitive emergency system that triggers a 'fight or flight' response when we are facing danger or feeling exceptionally stressed by worries. Often relaxation and breathing techniques have the reverse effect, calming our minds and bodies. Try breathing in slowly to the count of four, and out to the count of five, while saying the word 'Trust'. Another effective physical tool can be to lie on the sofa and, starting from the toes, tense, hold and then relax every muscle right up to your face.

This may all sound disconnected from your current concerns, but how we feel affects the way we think, and how we think affects the way we feel. These tools and others can help to interrupt the worry cycle that can so often spiral out of control in pregnancy.[7]

### 4. Notice your dreams

As I conclude this chapter, a final something for you to reflect on in the coming weeks: your dreams. Pregnant women often sleep lightly towards the end of a pregnancy, and concerns or issues stirring within you may well be raised through dreams. Of course your dreams may not be significant at all, but the Bible is clear that God can speak to us through them.[8] As a parent-to-be, there can be so much change to process that some of it may appear in our dreams and daydreams.

During my pregnancy I had Christian counselling, which I had actually booked prior to discovering I was expecting. Few people have a chance to talk through in great detail all that is going on during this time in their lives, and I am hugely grateful that I had the opportunity to do so. In fact, had I not, this book might never have been written, for it was during the hours spent talking about what was going on in my head in the build-up to having a child that I realized just how much there is to work through. The timing can only have been God's. I spent a good few hours during the sessions discussing my prenatal dreams. I encourage you to give credence to yours, and explore them in thought and prayer.

The psalmist reminds us in Psalm 139 that God knows and cares even about your deepest thoughts and dreams – a comforting thought during a time when we can so easily feel exposed and vulnerable:

> O LORD, you have searched me
>    and you know me.
> You know when I sit and when I rise;
>    you perceive my thoughts from afar.
> You discern my going out and my lying down;
>    you are familiar with all my ways.
> (Psalm 139:1–3)

Why not commit your fears – whether easily acknowledged or surfacing in your dreams – to God now? Ask him to help you overcome them by his power. As you face some of your fears now, remember the promise in Deuteronomy 31:8: 'The LORD himself goes before you and will be with you; he will never leave you nor forsake you. Do not be afraid; do not be discouraged.'

## For reflection or discussion

1. What has been your greatest fear during pregnancy so far?
2. How do you tend instinctively to respond to your fears?
3. What practical tools have you learned to help overcome worries?

4.  Spend some time speaking out your worries to God
    and thanking him for the good things in your life at the
    moment.

# PART II: A NEW FAMILY

## 4. WHEN TWO BECOME THREE: STARTING A FAMILY

**By Louie**

I recently attended a wedding with a glaring omission. The enormous metaphorical elephant in the room was a deliberate avoidance of the subject of children.

Was it that to pray that the couple would one day have a family would be insensitive if they then found themselves unable to conceive? Surely that would be to deny the power of prayer? Or has choosing to be childless become such a real possibility – even for a Christian couple – that now to mention the topic in a wedding service would be to make an unfair assumption? Perhaps someone was worried that if children were mentioned, the bride might feel like she was about to become nothing more than a baby-rearing machine. Of course there may have been other sensitive issues at stake, accounting for why children were not mentioned.

In our culture, deciding not to have children – and aborting the 'inconvenient' ones – is fast becoming as normal as choosing to become a parent. But the Bible is clear that

children are a gift and a huge blessing, as we saw in some of
the passages we looked at in Chapter 1. Psalm 127 reminds
us of this:

> Sons are a heritage from the LORD,
>     children a reward from him.
> Like arrows in the hands of a warrior
>     are sons born in one's youth.
> Blessed is the man
>     whose quiver is full of them.
> (Psalm 127:3–5)

Back to the subject of weddings. Just as a marriage is for
life and not simply about your wedding day – so the goal
of your pregnancy is not just the birth. When my friend Ali
was expecting her first baby, she spent hours reading about
pregnancy. As the most clued-up mum-to-be ever, it didn't
surprise me that she had the smooth-running water birth
that I could only hope for! But when she got her baby home
from hospital she felt utterly helpless – she had thought only
as far ahead as the birth. She hadn't read a thing about how
to care for a baby. As you approach parenthood, I encourage
you to think beyond the imminent arrival of your new baby.
Allow yourself some space to dwell on the reality that you
are soon to start a new family.

### Family lasts for life

When we become parents, we create a new family unit that
will last for life. Before your baby is born, this can seem a
terrifying, and even a trapping prospect. But God planned
pregnancy as nine months (or 280 days – whichever sounds
longest to you!) for good reason, aside from the biological
ones. It gives us a really decent chunk of time in which to get

ready, not only to care for a baby, but also to become part
of a family.

So how can you prepare for the lifelong commitment of
raising children? In Luke 1:24 we read that Elizabeth took five
months in seclusion after becoming pregnant. Speculation
surrounds the reason for her taking this time out – but the
likelihood is that she was spending quality time with God
and making herself ready to become a parent. Popping off
for a five-month silent retreat may not be practical for you
or me during pregnancy. But Elizabeth's dedication to the
cause of becoming a mother lays down a challenge for us:
are we willing to let God mould and shape us in readiness
for becoming a parent? Many church leaders advise engaged
couples actively to prepare for marriage: are you ready to be
just as proactive in getting ready for this major life change?

As I mentioned in the previous chapter, during my pregnancy I attended counselling. Many of the reflections in the
latter part of this chapter come from my own explorations
of what it means to become a parent, made within that
context.

## Family in the Bible
It may be that your own childhood experience of being
family was a mixed, or even a deeply negative one. So while
you may want to provide your child with a loving and
healthy family environment in which to grow up, you might
wonder what this looks like in practice. The Bible's model of
family is a great place to start. I'm going to look at a few of its
strongest families to see what God's view of family is.

### Abraham and his expansive family
God's call to Abraham shows the opportunity and blessing
that family can be. God says to him, 'Leave your country,

your people and your father's household and go to the land I will show you.' God says that if Abraham will do this:

> I [God] will make you into a great nation
>> and I will bless you;
> I will make your name great . . .
> (Genesis 12:1–2)

God then makes a covenant promise with Abraham, recorded in Genesis 17. And it's here that Abraham, who was previously called Abram, is given a significant new name by God. His new name Abraham means 'father of many'. God says:

> No longer will you be called Abram; your name will be Abraham, for I have made you a father of many nations. I will make you very fruitful; I will make nations of you, and kings will come from you. I will establish my covenant as an everlasting covenant between me and you and your descendants after you for the generations to come, to be your God and the God of your descendants after you.
> (Genesis 17:5–7)

If Abraham would worship God, prioritizing him even above his own family, he would in turn be blessed with children, grandchildren, great-grandchildren and more! His family would have the privilege of owning the land of Canaan and would become the founding tribe of the nation of Israel. When Jesus came to earth, it was as a descendant of Abraham (see Matthew 1), showing that family is God's chosen vehicle for bringing salvation to the world. As you start your own family, have you thought about the possibility of your passing on godliness to your children, and one day, to your children's children too?

Although I was blessed to be brought up in a loving Christian family, I still needed to reflect on Abraham's story with its message that God is passionate about using family, before starting to become excited about having a family of my own. With lots of single and married-but-childless friends, it was easy to assume that having a child would mean stress and hassle: sleepless nights, smelly nappies and having to socialize with strange eco-mother types. Before you have kids, you can be unaware of the fun and joy in parenting, which makes all those other things worth the effort. Do you need God to etch on your heart that there is real kingdom significance in the step you are taking?

### Ruth: *rewarded for her commitment to family*

The story of Ruth illustrates that God is pleased with you as you set out to start a family. Despite her tough circumstances, Ruth is committed to family in an astounding way and God richly blesses her as a result. Most married women expect a few rocky times in their relationship with their mother-in-law, but in Ruth's case it's within this very relationship that intense love for, and loyalty to, family is demonstrated (see Ruth 1 – 4).

Ruth's impassioned speech to Naomi shows how highly she esteems the bond of family:

> Don't urge me to leave you or to turn back from you. Where you go I will go, and where you stay I will stay. Your people will be my people and your God my God. Where you die I will die, and there I will be buried. May the LORD deal with me, be it ever so severely, if anything but death separates you and me.
>
> (Ruth 1:16–17)

God rewards Ruth for her costly obedience to him with a marriage proposal from Boaz. The woman who

honoured God by putting family first is blessed with a new
family. As the story is wrapped up, both she and Naomi
have a secure future ahead of them, and Ruth has a son
(Ruth 4:13).

Nicky, mum to twins, Felicity and Juliette, two, commented to us on the cost of becoming a parent: 'Your own
needs kind of go out of the window the second you become
a mother. Your baby always takes priority. But funnily
enough, you don't seem to mind very much.' When we had
Skye, the need to sacrifice for her suddenly became real.
Ruth's story gives me comfort that the sacrifices we make as
parents are worthwhile.

### Cornelius and Lydia: invite their families to meet God

Sharing the message of Jesus with people who don't yet know
him is a priority for Will and me. The stories of Cornelius
and Lydia found in the book of Acts can inspire parents-to-
be regarding the potential for friendship evangelism in the
context of new parenthood. Their stories show how God is
often discovered in and through family. We are finding that
starting a family opens new doors to sharing Christ, not only
with your own children, but also with the other families you
will soon be spending more time with.

Cornelius, along with his family, is a devout and God-
fearing Gentile (Acts 10:1–2). He would not have known the
truth of who Jesus was, however. One day an angel appears
to him when he is praying, commanding him to invite the
apostle Peter to his house. No doubt risking his reputation
among his friends, family and wider group of relatives,
Cornelius makes the bold move of inviting all of them to
his home to listen to Peter tell them about Jesus. The Holy
Spirit falls on the group as Peter speaks, and they convert to
become followers of Christ. Thanks to Cornelius' willingness

to bring his family to God, a huge group of people discover Christ for the first time.

A similar pattern is repeated with Lydia, a successful businesswoman whom we come across later in Acts. Lydia probably had a big family, large home and heaps of servants. When she finds faith in God, she has her whole household baptized along with her (Acts 16:13–15). Fearless of spreading the good news, Lydia, like Cornelius, recognizes family as the most important place to bring Jesus into.

## Value your values
Our quick zoom around some of the families in the Bible brings to light some relieving truths: there's no biblical blueprint for how to be the perfect parent, and there's no blueprint for just what an 'ideal' family looks like either. Indeed the perfect family just doesn't exist!

A look at some of the families in the Bible does teach us, however, that the values we hold as parents – and which we consequently pass on to our children – are what bring shape and identity to our particular family. The first months or even years of being a parent may be very practical in focus, but the values we uphold will affect our approach from the start.

Lindsay and Mark Melluish write in their book *Family Time*:

> It is very easy to head out into family life without knowing which way we are going. But how much better to have a destination in mind and to feel secure in where we are heading . . .
>
> That end destination will shape the values we have in our family, and those values will shape the way in which we work as a family in the here and now. They will give our family its individual feel – its DNA.[1]

During the summer that I was pregnant, Will and I attended a condensed version of The Parenting Course run by Nicky and Sila Lee.[2] One of their exercises challenged us to think constructively about the values that we as parents would like to give our children. They asked us, 'When your children are eighteen and look back on their childhood, what values will stand out as having been essential to their upbringing?'

Will and I later discussed this together, trying to pin down a set of values pleasing to God that we would want our children to absorb throughout childhood. Seeing love modelled in our relationship and knowing that they are loved were at the top of our list. Being accepted just as they are (regardless of what they do or don't do) and praying as a family were also priorities, as were talking openly, laughing and having fun together.

Your list may look very different from ours, and that's fine. I suggest you write your list on paper and pray it through. I'm expecting to come back to that list at some really challenging times in the future.

### Your childhood values

Have you tried answering the question we looked at in the section above, in relation to your own childhood experience? If you want to try this now, here's the question rephrased for you: 'When you look back at your own childhood, what values stand out as having been essential in your family and upbringing?'

You may already have spent time thinking through the values you imbibed from your parents, and the ways that your wider family still operates today, especially if you previously did marriage preparation or had counselling. You are likely to have decided which values you respect and want to emulate in your own relationship or family, and which ones you want to leave behind. If this is an area that you haven't yet explored, I encourage you to look at it with your spouse during pregnancy. Will helps you begin to do so in the next chapter.

## Your current relational situation

To what extent have you thought about your own family relationships and how these might be affected by your new arrival? You may find that, as you progress through this season, your thinking on these things is changing too. As my pregnancy drew towards its end, I increasingly had the sense that I was representing both myself and our baby. This changed the dynamic in conversations with Will.

Here are some questions and issues to consider.

### 1. How will having a baby change your relationship with your parents?

I found that during my pregnancy, my mother and I spent more time talking than ever before. I think the connection between us increased because we had something new and deeply significant in common – she had given birth and raised children and now her own daughter was going to do so too.

She and I are very practical people and, while I was pregnant, my parents borrowed or bought just about every piece of equipment needed for a new baby – so that we would have everything we needed for the baby when we went to stay with them. Much as I was grateful, I found this overwhelming – I hadn't even had the baby yet! I was also aware that once I had my baby, my relationship with my mother could easily become focused purely on childcare and not move into healthy communication about ourselves or our feelings.

As you think about how bringing a baby into the world

will affect your relationship with your parents, you may want to consider the possible effects of the change on other family members too. If your parents are divorced or remarried, you may also have a different family dynamic to think about.

### 2. What sort of relationship does your spouse have with his/her parents? How might this be affected by him/her becoming a parent?

Just as your own relationship with your parents will change to some extent when you have a child, remember that your spouse will face this with his/her parents too. These changes are likely to affect you. This makes it all the more important that, during pregnancy, both you and your spouse work on your relationship with your respective families, thinking particularly about how you communicate with them. We agreed early on in our marriage to try our very best not to be offended when one of us found our in-laws frustrating or difficult to understand. This has been hugely helpful in our discussions about our respective families, especially during pregnancy, and has helped us to try to see each other's perspectives without being insulted by them.

Hard as these discussions may be, they are worth the effort. A family's heritage is often passed down through the generations. This is true not only in the spiritual sense, but also in terms of how we interact and communicate. Unhealthy patterns of family interaction that can be broken and changed now will help to provide a more stable relational environment for your child to enter into.

### 3. What sort of role do you expect the grandparents to take?

If your parents are becoming grandparents for the first time, spare them a compassionate thought – they are probably feeling just as nervous about their new role as you are! One of our relatives recently went on a course in 'how to be a good grandparent'. While my mother didn't attend such a course, she certainly expressed the fact that she was a bit unsure at first of just how to fill her new granny shoes!

Rachel Waddilove, a grandmother, writes in *The Baby Book*,

> One of the most challenging things as a grandparent is realizing that your children and their partners are a new family unit who need your respect. It can be tempting to give your own children advice, forgetting that they are now the parents, not you . . .
>
> Often a son-in-law can feel very pushed out and resentful of his mother-in-law, particularly if she 'takes over' with the baby or outstays her welcome. Daughters-in-law often struggle with how to include both their parents and in-laws, and as grandparents it's important to be able to stand back and not add to the pressure.[3]

If you have strong feelings about the sort of role you want your parents to take when they become grandparents, it may be wise to discuss this together before the baby arrives. This can help avoid potential disappointment or annoyance from both sides of the fence. You may simply want to agree that you will talk about this with them in the future, when you have more of an idea of what could work for you all.

Think too about how your parents might be in the presence of a baby. Will they struggle to know how to interact or be natural? This may give you an indicator of how they were with you as a child, which in turn can help you understand some of the ways in which you yourself were parented.

As you consider the role you hope your own parents to take in your lives when the baby arrives, it's also worth thinking specifically about their part in the birth and the very early days. When my Hindu friend Rakhi gave birth, her mother was her birthing partner. Rakhi got back from hospital to receive six weeks of dedicated care from her mother-in-law. During those weeks, Rakhi was not allowed out of the house, all her food was cooked in ghee, and her local friends and family constantly dropped in to help in the house – and no doubt coo over the baby too.

When your baby is born, who do you hope to do what, and when? Avoiding making assumptions about your parents' part in these details can help your birth pan out more smoothly.

**What's your advice on dealing with your parents and in-laws in the first few months of being a parent?**

'Accept all the help that they offer, and be very grateful. Remember that, although you want time alone with your baby, which you are obviously totally entitled to, this is their grandchild whom they love almost as much as you do. Let them have special time with the baby, and use that time to sleep or relax.' Nicky, mum to twins Felicity and Juliette, two

'All parents try to offer advice on various aspects of parenting, usually starting with, "We didn't have those when you were young. We used to . . ." My advice is to listen as sometimes it turns out to be useful! Be clear in setting the boundaries, however, and push back if you don't agree – it's your family and your baby.' Chris, dad to Harry, eighteen months

'I think mums and mums-in-law are surprised by how

strongly they feel about the baby. My mum says she feels the same about her grandchildren as she does about my brother and me. At times you have to remind them kindly that they are not your child's mother.' Tilly, mum to Naomi, four, and Sebastian, two

## 4. How is your marriage?

When did you and your spouse last sit down and have an honest chat about how your marriage is going? In the final weeks of my pregnancy I often felt tired and grumpy, and the last thing I wanted to do was intentionally work on our relationship. In retrospect, I wish we had carved out more special time together in those final pre-baby weeks. Try to make the most of your time off together and invest as much as you can in your marriage. It wasn't until five weeks after the birth of our daughter that Will and I finally had the time – or were sufficiently awake – to communicate properly about our relationship and how we were dealing with the huge challenge of caring for our new family member.

Before our daughter was born, we decided we would take what I like to call 'a marriage-centred approach' to parenting. We believe that the love modelled between a child's parents has a more significant effect on his or her development than the practical ways in which they care for their child. In fact, the latter flows from the former.

The love you model within your own relationship as parents will provide normality and a peaceful home envi-ronment for your child to grow up in. In *The Parenting Book*, Nicky and Sila Lee write,

A strong, loving relationship between us as parents is one of the greatest gifts we can give to our children. The knowledge that we will stay together through thick and thin, working through difficulties and resolving disagreements, gives our children a deep sense of security . . .

They observe how we speak to each other: whether we listen or make demands, whether we are rude or show respect, whether we are appreciative or critical of each other. They notice the physical contact, or lack of it, between us. They see how we express our anger and watch how we resolve conflict. They take in whether we apologise or never admit to being wrong, whether we hold grudges or forgive each other.

Our marriage acts as a role model for our children and for their relationships.[4]

As I write this chapter, it is seven weeks since Skye's birth, and I'm beginning to realize just what a challenge it is to be committed to marriage-centred parenting. But I'm determined we will stick to it! Doing so means making some practical decisions to ensure that love flows in your relationship and you don't become two child carers who eat and sleep in the same house, but no longer invest in each other. We plan to restart having a regular marriage time together as soon as our daughter is old enough for a babysitter. Until then we're focusing on snatching even the smallest of quality moments to hang out together, pray for a few minutes for each other before Will heads off to work, or go for a walk and talk while Skye is sleeping in the buggy. Thinking about how you might work these sorts of marriage-building moments into your day with a baby around is worth doing now – creative thinking happens at a slower pace when you're sleep deprived!

## How do you maintain a good marriage when a baby comes on the scene?

'Expect that the first couple of months will be given over to living day by day, with the joys, challenges and tiredness that come with having a baby. I think our marriage was sustained by going for walks with Amelie in a carry sling – she was quiet and we could chat. Incorporating marriage time into the everyday chores is critical.' Alise, mum to Amelie, six, and Isaac, five

'Talking as often as possible and working out what each other needs – perhaps distraction, a break, seeing friends, time alone or time together – is so important. One of the things we learned is to try to steer clear of drifting from one day to the next. This can get really depressing if all you can see before you is days and days of looking after the baby. Planning time off, or adventures with or without your baby, breaks up the routine and helps the marriage so much.' Tom, dad to April, six months

'A lot of people talk about the early weeks as being a particularly taxing time in your marriage but I didn't find that they were. Sure, tiredness can turn the happiest camper into a raving loony – but as long as your husband is understanding and appreciates that this behaviour is only temporary, then I think having a baby brings a husband and wife closer together.' Nicky, mum to twins Felicity and Juliette, two

## 5. Your new trio

When you move from being a couple to becoming a family of three, everyone's roles get shaken up. Adding a third person to your family unit can create tension, even if he or she is welcome. Naomi Stadlen writes,

> A two-person relationship is dramatically different from one of three people. A two-person relationship has a kind of elegant symmetry, whereas this three-person one is complex ... the three-person relationship can operate as three separate individuals, or one set of three people or three sets of pairs ...[5]

Both Will and I had to work through the almost jealous feelings that come when your spouse seems to have a new number one to care for. Initially, in some ways our daughter felt like a competitor to our relationship. I now realize that my love for Skye can be just as strong as my love for Will, without the two conflicting, because they are such different relationships. However in the early weeks, a father often struggles to understand his place, as mum is primary caregiver and dad feels left out. Once we had talked about this, we tried to ensure that the love flowed three ways between us. I encouraged Will to spend lots of time cuddling and playing with Skye; I wanted to avoid any competition between us for her love or attention, or her building a bond with me alone.

Will further explores changes to your relationships as a new parent in Chapter 8. In the meantime, have you considered the day-to-day adjustments you may need to make as a couple, in order to embrace a new rhythm of life as a trio? As you reflect on this, you may like to think about our triune God, who demonstrates perfect love flowing between three separate and distinct, and yet wholly united, individuals.

## For reflection or discussion

1. Are you excited about starting a family? If not, ask God why this might be.
2. How willing are you for God to use your new family to build his kingdom? How might you envisage him doing this?
3. Return to the question about developing family values on page 78. Discuss this with your spouse and come up with your own list.
4. Talk about how you plan to maintain a strong marriage during the first few months of parenthood.

## 5. WHAT IF WE END UP LIKE OUR PARENTS? DEALING WITH FAMILY DAMAGE

**By Will**

I've been asked the question in the title of this chapter by many young couples preparing for marriage. In a generation where growing up with divorced parents is a common experience – and a quarter of families in the UK are headed up by a lone parent – the fear of repeating the mistakes of older generations is prevalent. My advice has always been that we cannot shape our lives around what we are not, but only around what we are. The reality is that every couple will at some point show similarities to their parents' relationships – even if those relationships are not ones we hoped to emulate. We cannot escape the reality that our upbringing, experiences, values and even our genetics have a part to play in the people we have become.

In some traditions, Christians have imbibed unhelpful theological emphases that suggest that it is possible to deny the impact of our familial heritage. Of course the power of the gospel is that we can be freed from past sin, and even healed from damage that others have done to us. But the gospel is about redemption and not about erasing our history, no matter how uncomfortable or unhappy it might have been. With this in mind, we need to try to approach parenting, not from a context of neutrality, but from a realistic view of how we ourselves were parented.

In the previous chapter, Louie introduced the idea of spending time reflecting on your own childhood as a way of becoming more aware of the influences that have shaped us. Danny Silk writes, 'The question we all need to ask is, "What did I learn to be true in childhood, and are those beliefs really the truth?" This will help us identify the truth that we are instilling in the hearts of our own children.'[1] In this chapter I will help you further to explore your own upbringing in preparation for parenthood.

## How were you brought up?

As we reflect on our upbringing, some of us idealize the experience but others 'catastrophize' it (sometimes for good reason). Try to look back at how you were raised with as much objectivity as you can muster. The likelihood is that there are aspects of your childhood that you recall with a smile, and there are also ways in which your family operated that you are not keen to replicate. It is important to note that nobody was raised perfectly, but fortunately few people have had a completely negative experience either.

If you are coming to parenting as a couple, you will be bringing two sets of perhaps very different experiences to the cradle of your new baby. It is essential that, while you might be unified on which of your own parents did the 'best' job, you do not fall into the trap of believing that you should or could just follow their example yourselves. One mum-to-be in week thirty-six of pregnancy commented, 'The practicalities of parenthood and raising a child still seem a long way off. I imagine that, when I get there, I'll automatically adopt some of the same principles and parenting skills that my parents used. I hope my husband and I will learn along the way and cross each bridge as we come to it.'

Simply copying the approach of one set of parents may appear to be an easy option, but it is problematic for a number of reasons. The first is that any particular parenting model isn't perfect – it is just comparably better than another approach. The second is that, if you prioritize one partner's parenting model over another, when things don't go according to plan there is the potential to lay blame or absolve oneself of responsibility. The third issue is that, while we may think we are parenting to choice, we will still, to some extent, be unconsciously enacting our own upbringing experiences.

## Unconscious drivers

As this is a book about preparing for parenthood, and not so much about how to parent, I hope to focus in this chapter predominantly upon this third issue: the unconscious drivers that we first bring to parenthood.

In my work on emotional health within churches, I sometimes ask a congregation, 'How many people use the gym?' Generally lots of hands go up. Then I ask, 'And who regularly thinks about their health?' Again, thinking about how to stay well is on most people's agendas. My next question is, 'How many people think about their thinking?' I'm discovering a pattern: most people think about their overall health and fitness, and many do something about it by exercising regularly. But few of us think about what we think about! We consider our thinking as something automatic and non-moveable. Yet, how we think is, in fact, the lens by which we view everything else, therefore it has a huge bearing on the choices we make. Examining the way we view the past, or the way we tend to think about the future, can lead us to make healthier and more objective decisions.

## Solid foundations

Jesus taught a parable about two builders who started from different positions. One began to build his house upon sand and the other built upon rock.

Jesus said:

> Therefore everyone who hears these words of mine and puts them into practice is like a wise man who built his house on the rock. The rain came down, the streams rose, and the winds blew and beat against that house; yet it did not fall, because it had its foundation on the rock. But everyone who hears these words of mine and does not put them into practice is like a foolish man who built his house on sand. The rain came down, the streams rose, and the winds blew and beat against that house, and it fell with a great crash.
>
> (Matthew 7:24–27)

I am sure that both builders in the story wanted to create fantastic houses, but intentions aside, it was the foundations on which they built that determined the strength (or lack of it) of the houses they ended up with. Jesus makes the point here that we are to build our lives – and our family – upon him. He is the only sure foundation.

We may feel that we cannot choose the foundation materials that we bring to parenting, because we sense we are purely the product of our own experiences of being parented. But the great news is that, as Christians, we aren't left in a position of choiceless inevitability. Jesus can heal and restore even the most broken foundations. What we need to do in preparation for parenthood is become aware of the foundation material already laid down in our lives, prayerfully asking God in what areas we need to seek his restoration.

## Reacting against your own upbringing

### Geoff and Lindsey's story

As a young child, Geoff attended a boys' private school in the hills of North Wales. On the rare occasions that his father came to collect him at the end of term, they would shake hands formally in front of the car. Geoff could see other children being kissed and hugged by their parents, but not him. Geoff's memories of early childhood were marked by the need for discipline and acceptable behaviour. When he went off to university, his behaviour initially became wild. But he was quickly drawn to the message of Jesus' love and acceptance as something he had never known personally. Geoff became a Christian before leaving university, and a few years later he met and married Lindsey. They subsequently found out that she was pregnant.

As Geoff and Lindsey prepared for the birth, they had some heated arguments. Neither could understand why there was such tension in the air, but every time they discussed potential baby routines, Geoff would get angry or go off in a sulk. Lindsey had no idea why he was so determined that they go down the demand-feeding route, or why he seemed to want to sabotage her attempts to plan structure into their child's life. Geoff felt passionate about what he didn't want them to do, but equally felt apathetic about the alternatives. Neither Geoff nor Lindsey could understand why this apparently small issue was stealing so much of their joy and excitement about the imminent birth of their first child.

Reaction formation is an extremely common human phenomenon. If we are stung by a bee, we formulate a reaction to all bees which encourages caution and distance. If we didn't react to negative or potentially threatening experiences, we would keep on getting stung or hurt. While reaction formation is therefore usually very useful, at times it can be unhealthy. Geoff had not experienced a natural form of danger like a bee sting, but he had suffered from an emotionally absent parenting style that left him feeling unloved. It doesn't take a genius to see how his childhood experiences informed his decision-making about the way he wanted to raise their child.

I hope that this example scenario helps to illuminate that we are not 'neutral', but bring our own experiences into our parenting. If we were to ask Geoff what he wants for his unborn child, I think he would say, 'I want him or her to feel really loved.' Of course this is exactly the right thing to hope for, but the only difficulty is that Geoff has equated structured parenting models with coldness and distance. By making this connection, Geoff is assuming that flexibility and love go together and that order is paired with a lack of emotion. The reality is that neither structured nor flexible parenting models actually determine whether a child feels loved or not.

Geoff and Lindsey would do well to discuss their own experiences of being parented and ask each other which memories provoke particularly strong feelings within them. They may then be able to understand where the connections are being made in their own approach to parenting, and choose a style that is not reactive but appropriate.

The celebrity chef and author Nigella Lawson's reflections on her upbringing and her love of baking offer another example of reaction formation. In *How to Eat*, she writes about how her mother and grandmother never made sweet things. As a result, Nigella lacked confidence in her own ability to bake. When she had her own children, baking cupcakes with them was an activity she relished, and Nigella is probably now best known for her incredible cake and pudding recipes. Gilly Smith writes in her biography of the chef, '*How to be a Domestic Goddess* is a homage to her inner pastry chef, claiming the smells and tastes that were never developed at her mother's side.'[2] In an interview, Nigella said, 'Perhaps making cupcakes is an idealised version of a childhood I didn't have.'[3]

As Christians we trust in a God of redemption who can lead us to become parents who provide love and stability for our own families. The gospel is powerful to transform, but sometimes we need to face the past in order to allow its power to infiltrate those memories and stop them from leading us towards distorted reactions. I have always admired my own mother's ability to parent with real compassion and openness, despite the more distant parenting she received as she grew up. Her experience of knowing Jesus' love has kept her own heart soft and warm, where others might have become closed off. Her example challenges me: am I willing to usher the presence of Jesus into my past, allowing the Holy Spirit to prompt me towards forgiveness, acceptance and peace? If we do this, the foundations of our parenting are more likely to be built on the rock of Jesus than on the sands of our brokenness.

## Enid Blyton experiences

Some prospective parents have the opposite reaction to Geoff: we review our childhood through unduly rosy spectacles. While training for ministry, I worked for a few months as an assistant chaplain in a senile dementia unit in Oxford.

This was one of the most wonderful and formative ministry experiences for me, but I spent a lot of time talking about the 'good ol' days' with the patients. As they perused the newspapers, they would tut with dismay, and then tell me about their childhoods. With surprising uniformity, everything was once better, brighter, safer and more innocent – despite the fact that many of them had lived through two world wars, Spanish flu, the Great Depression and many other global catastrophes.

We all have the propensity to filter our memories. In fact this is precisely what we spend a lot of our lives doing. Generally we try to forget the bad and remember the good. We have a conscious selection of memories that we hold on to because they have particular significance for us. When we consider our own childhood, some of us will hold on to a distorted selection of negative memories, some have a range that is balanced, and others will have filtered out all of their negative experiences altogether. This can leave an individual with a sense that their childhood was uniquely wonderful, akin to an Enid Blyton novel, with endless lashings of ginger beer and ham sandwiches eaten on picnics in the shade of the magical faraway tree.

So why do we filter our memories like this? Sometimes it is because we want to protect an image of our parents and hold on to them as the perfect ideal. Sometimes it is because we have actually had some bad experiences in childhood that we don't want to face, so we create a perfect picture of childhood to blot them out. Another common motive for idealization is that our current life is unpredictable or threatening, so we create a safe haven of good childhood memories. Then when things in life feel too difficult, we can retreat into that historic comfort blanket.

## Lara and Oliver's story

Lara was from a small town in New Jersey and had first come to the UK on a student exchange programme. Here she met an Englishman whom she subsequently married. Oliver came from a more turbulent family background and, while his parents were still together, there was a lot of tension between them. The first few years of marriage were comfortable, but Oliver had a tendency to get drawn into his work and neglect Lara's emotional needs. Having already made the difficult cultural transition to the UK from the US, Lara was vulnerable to fantasizing about home, family and friends. She missed the beautiful fall season, her parents' easy demeanour and the structure of her old life.

Lara found out that she was pregnant during an exceptionally busy period in Oliver's work. While he was over the moon about the baby, he left her to begin the process of preparation for parenthood unsupported. The daunting distance from home seemed even greater now that she was pregnant, and Lara began to communicate with her parents every day, seeking their support and comfort.

When Oliver's project calmed down, he began to engage Lara in conversations about how they would bring up their child. Every time he would make a suggestion, Lara would begin to reminisce about her own upbringing, how perfect her own parents were, and why they should do exactly the same as her parents had done for their own child. Every time he made a suggestion, she would be disparaging about the state of his parents' relationship and dismiss it out of hand. As Lara spent more and more time on the phone home, Oliver began to despair about his own role as a father.

I hope that this illustration shows the negative impact that a distorted, over-positive view of our childhood experiences can have. Jesus has called us to be children of the light, who live by the truth. Any distortion of the truth is a lie and has no place in the foundations of our family. In this instance, Lara's distorted view brought her comfort and security, but ultimately it drove a wedge between her and her husband as they prepared for the birth of their child. The couple needed to review their experiences and look for value in both. Then they needed to pray about how they would approach parenting.

**Do you tend to idealize or criticize the way you were raised?**

'Where do I start? There is very little that I received from my father that I would like to emulate. I strive to be all that he wasn't, while being aware that I don't want to act unhealthily out of this brokenness.' Paul, dad to Sam, five, Owen, four and Hope, one

'I probably do a mixture of the two. My mum was awesome with us as babies. I'm one of five, and she certainly seemed to revel in the "young children phase" and did an amazing job of it. She was loving, selfless and completely tireless in her energy for us. So, in terms of how I approach this current stage, I feel I have a terrific role model that I will try my best to live up to. My teen years were a different story – I was pretty unhappy and rebellious and don't think either of my parents dealt well with that.' Ellen, mum to April, six months

'As new parents, it's hard not to think: here's a clean slate and, with the right approach, we can discourage swearing, eating too much sugar or watching too much TV. But then something happens that helps you understand, or if necessary forgive, your parents' attitude to childrearing: you realize parenting is a long slog. You start out really enthusiastic, but sometimes you're just empty or tired and you can't fight another battle, so you compromise on something you thought you wouldn't. It sounds obvious, but it only makes sense when you have a child of your own.' Andrew, dad to Jack, eight weeks

## What about generational patterns?

Many people have to endure significant challenge or pain as children. There are also some families in which a generational history of family issues such as alcoholism, abuse, eating disorders, psychological breakdown or suicide can be traced. If this is true of your family, having a child may provoke deep fears. You may feel anxious that you are being reckless by bringing someone new into the world. You may fear that, given your family history, it is inevitable that you will fail to be a good parent, and the same generational behaviour will pass through you to your child.

Before we look at these issues in more detail, I want to reiterate that nothing is inevitable where God is concerned. He can and will break the power of the past over your life and your future. Jesus' work on the cross means that even the most entrenched patterns of behaviour can be broken and that we can have a new start as parents-to-be. Thinking about some of these things can seem frightening, but try not to be afraid. It may be that, for you, bringing some of the past to mind is bringing it to the foot of the cross. When we can see patterns and pitfalls for what they are, we can pray about them and bring them under Jesus' authority.

If you read the two Old Testament books of Kings, you can see several strong links between generations of leaders. 1 Kings 15:3 says of Abijah, 'He committed all the sins his father had done before him; his heart was not fully devoted to the LORD his God . . .' Often, what is modelled by a father to his son leads to similar behaviours and outlooks in the next generation. As parents we need to recognize the incredible power of behavioural modelling. Tim, dad to Ridley, thirteen months, and Bethan, one week, said of behavioural modelling as a new parent, 'You have to be aware that how you act and behave is being viewed and monitored by little eyes. You are shaping what he will become.'

There are several kings who break the mould, and operate in a different way from their parents.[4] They are proof that, despite the most entrenched familial patterns, God can intervene. No-one is predestined to a life of brokenness because of their background. However, we also know that the propensity for these negative strands to replicate within subsequent generations is high if no direct and deliberate action is taken.

## Three ways to take action

What then can we do when we fear that history may repeat itself? The first thing is to approach things in the spiritual realm. Within my work among people with addictions and emotional disturbances, I have seen that where there is a spiritual root to a problem, no amount of practical or emotional support can alone bring about change. But where a spiritual foundation is broken, practical and emotional work can begin to have an impact. In Matthew 18:18 Jesus teaches his disciples about the principles of binding and loosing. He says, 'I tell you the truth, whatever you bind on earth will be bound in heaven, and whatever you loose on earth will be loosed in heaven.' We too can pray as Jesus teaches the disciples to do here: binding in his name behavioural patterns we feel have a spiritual hold within our family relationships. Prayers in the name of Jesus bring freedom in the earthly and spiritual realms.

### 1. Pray with others

If you can see strong generational patterns of abuse, addictions, abandonment, conflict or anything else negative, then you need to pray this through with a trusted friend or spiritual mentor. I suggest that you list the generational patterns you are aware of, and also the things that you most fear will impact on your own child. In Jesus' name bind those things that have influenced your family historically and pray for a loosing of binding fears. While praying, be open to anything that the Holy Sprit may bring to mind, vocalize it and pray it through.

Dealing with the spiritual requires faith that, once you have brought these things to Jesus, he has dealt with them. It is important that, having dealt with things in the spiritual realm, you then continue to face up to them in emotional and practical ways.

### 2. Get practical

Even when we have dealt with things in the spiritual realm, individuals may still have a place of weakness common to their family, meaning that, while failure is not inevitable, practical steps must be taken to safeguard their family's future. For instance, 50% of today's alcoholics also had an alcoholic parent – the familial link is unequivocal. I am certain that not a single one of those parents intended for their addiction to influence their child, let alone for it to be manifest in that child when he or she grew up.

In Genesis 4:7 God says to Cain, 'Sin is crouching at your door; it desires to have you, but you must master it.' God's instruction to have mastery over sin is a practical one and requires a very practical response.

## Antley's story

One of my good friends, Antley, a church leader from Jacksonville, Florida says: 'I remember my childhood being filled with random, uncomfortable and often very confusing (and embarrassing) instances of my adoptive parents' behaviour when they had been drinking. The result was that I grew up in a very scary and unstable environment. Even though there was no physical or verbal abuse, the uncertainty of what awaited me at home caused patterns of fear and anxiety to follow me throughout my life. Because of their inability to function as my parents, I often found myself in situations where I had to "be the parent" and make decisions that they should have been making. This robbed me of my childhood, and the freedom that I should have had to play, risk and fail in a safe environment. Children need a family that will love and protect them regardless of their mistakes.

'When I was preparing to become a father, I became eager to meet my natural biological parents and find out what my medical history was. Upon meeting my birth mother, I was discouraged, but not surprised, to find out that she too was an alcoholic. With the growing responsibility of having children and providing for my own family, our relationship quickly dissolved when I chose not to "be the parent" in another dysfunctional relationship.

'As an adult, I did not drink frequently, but I displayed signs of over-drinking. From time to time I experienced blackouts and lied about how much I had had to drink. Concerned about this, I went to several counsellors, all of whom said I had nothing to fear, and that my over-reaction to my drinking patterns was due to my Christian convictions. Even with their understanding of my family history, their conclusions all supported that I did not have a drinking problem.

'However, when we were getting ready to have children, my wife and I decided that it was not worth the risk of putting our children through the same childhood circumstances that I had gone through, and we decided that I would not drink at all any more.

'When we made this decision, we told our small group and they began to pray that God would take away the desire I had to drink so that it would not be a struggle. That was my first experience of God doing a "miracle" in my life. The urge and desire to drink totally left me.

'We have four children now, three biological boys and an adopted little girl from Russia. All of them stretch my parenting skills and my patience. I am sure there will be other negative patterns and behaviours that I will pass on to my children. There are often times when I fail miserably as a parent, but what I know for sure is that the instability, fear and confusion created by alcoholism in my life will stop with me because of God's love for me, his forgiveness and his grace.'

Many Christians bring generational patterns under the power of the cross, but then abdicate their own responsibility for good decision-making from that point onwards. It is as if they are saying to God, 'I want you to do something about this, but I can't or won't.' It is essential if we are really taking God seriously – and taking parenting seriously – that our actions correlate with our beliefs. If you know that there have been generational patterns in your family, don't just say they will never happen to you: put practical safeguards in place to ensure that they don't.

A final important practical step is to consider seeking appropriate professional help and support in addressing these issues.

### 3. Face the emotional

I have left dealing with the emotional challenges presented by breaking generational patterns until last because it is often not as straightforward as taking prayerful or practical action. Impending parenthood definitely brings wider family relationships and history into view, and there is sometimes a significant emotional cost to admitting that all we see is not ideal.

I wonder if, when you think about the way you were raised, you feel a certain level of defensiveness about your parents' intentions, even if you know that they were less than perfect. I have often heard fathers advocating physical punishment for their own children on the basis that the physical treatment they endured did them 'no harm'. Sadly, the reality is often that for many individuals these physical punishments were abusive and damaging. Passing on such treatment can in some way actually be a defence of a parent's relationship with the grandparent. The parent may question the love that they were shown, but in an attempt to reassure themselves, they normalize that behaviour and pass it on. They may think, 'I know I love my child and so if I physically punish them, that shows that my dad also loved me, despite the fact that he punished me in that way.' Whether or not we should use physical punishment in child discipline is another debate and one that we do not have time to look into further here, but I hope this example serves to indicate how insecurities about our childhood relationships can be the driving force behind generational patterns.

Facing up to the emotional challenge of breaking generational patterns can be particularly hard, because it often means dealing with some of the deeper insecurities we have about our own experiences. Stopping these things from influencing our children means consciously deciding that there were things in our own upbringing that were not good, healthy or godly. This sort of consideration and objectivity may lead to surprising feelings of raw disappointment, anger or grief in your own heart. You may also feel that this is somewhat indulgent, given that this book is about preparing to be a parent yourself. However, I would say that the contrary is true. By having the courage to face up to some tough emotional issues, you are in fact preparing in the best possible way to become a parent yourself.

## Continue to develop your own self-awareness

Today I read *Kipper's A–Z* to Skye in bed at a very early hour of the morning. She wanted to grab each page and turn it, nearly always in the wrong direction! It would have been easier to go Z–A, and therein lies the truth I have been driving towards in this chapter. Parenting isn't neatly ordered; it is unpredictable. Despite what the books say, when your baby arrives, he or she won't begin at the beginning and neatly jump through different developmental hoops. And neither will you.

In my estimation, parenting is 20% knowledge and 80% instinct. While it may seem beneficial to glean all the knowledge you can, I think it is equally important to examine your instincts. We need regularly to ask ourselves why behaving in a certain way seems automatic to us. Or why we might find ourselves reacting so strongly to something we know could be viewed as a relatively small issue. I believe that, in preparation for parenthood, the creation of a broad foundation of self-awareness, confidence, reflection and prayer is fundamental to realizing our ultimate aim – that our child feels loved and secure. It is also nonsense to think that, by reading this book or doing some initial preparation, you have climbed the mountain. In fact, the continued process of emotional response, reflection and adaptation will be your bread and butter as a parent.

## For reflection or discussion

1. Take some time to talk through the highlights and lowlights of your childhood family experience with your spouse.
2. As you look back on your upbringing, do you have a tendency to be super-positive or super-negative?
3. How could you further develop your own levels of self-awareness?

# PART III: THE BIRTH

## 6. HAPPY BIRTHDAY: GIVING BIRTH WITH GOD ON SIDE

**By Louie**

I'm warning you now: this is the chapter on giving birth. If you're anything like I was at the start of my pregnancy, you will be skipping this chapter entirely. Until I was six months' pregnant I couldn't even bear thinking about giving birth: it terrified me.

As my pregnancy progressed, however, I became intrigued by what 'B-day' might entail. By month nine, however, I started to wonder if I had seen one too many graphic images of women popping out babies. I had read the birth sections of piles of pregnancy books, been to prenatal NCT classes and attended several talks at my hospital.

Unable to resist discovering more, one night when Will was out I sat down by myself to watch an NCT DVD of two women's birth stories. Watching such an unglamorous film of women going through the pain of childbirth – while knowing I might have to face something similar in just a matter of days – left me terrified all over again. I turned off my TV and sat in the quiet darkness of the empty house, shocked by what I'd just seen. It was time to trust God instead of relying on my own ability to prepare myself.

The balance between being reassuringly informed about what might happen when you give birth for the first time and not getting wound up by exposure to too many negative birth stories is a hard one to find. What I want to do in this chapter is share with you both my own and two other mothers' birth stories, as told in their own words. I aim to tell them with honesty and sensitivity.

Unlike what you might read or watch elsewhere, these are birth stories with God as a big part of the process. They are not here to frighten you – nor are they here to give you idealistic expectations of what giving birth is like. At times the stories in this and the following chapter may sound dramatic, but remember that the nature of giving birth for the first time is almost always dramatic and emotional, simply because of the magnitude of the event, however much the practicalities go according to plan.

## My own birth story: Skye

It was 3am on Christmas Eve. I had woken from a nightmare and my brain felt confused and fuzzy. I had been dreaming about tomorrow's Christmas lunch, when my parents were due to host twenty-five relatives for a huge festive roast. In my dream, I went into labour during the three-hour-long meal, during which I screamed from a bedroom, trying not to disrupt the party downstairs. When in reality the next day passed like any other family Christmas (bar the fact that I could hardly reach the table to eat due to the elephant-sized bump in my way), I breathed an enormous sigh of relief.

The build-up to Christmas had been vastly different from normal. I missed out on what seemed like tons of December parties because I was too exhausted to go out. I found myself at home on maternity leave instead, quietly reflecting on the life change ahead, watching mind-numbing daytime television and starting to write this book while bobbling on my birthing ball. (A birthing ball, by the way, is basically a gym ball. It's meant to make the baby get into the right position for giving birth, but I have no idea if it works or not.)

I had decided to stop work at thirty-five weeks, partly as I had sensed that God wanted me to be ready well before my due date. But the weeks rolled by and the baby showed no signs of coming whatsoever. I started to feel short-changed at the lack of baby appearance. Now, as I look back, I wonder whether God wanted me to take that extra time out before I had Skye, because mentally and emotionally I needed it to be ready for her.

With time on my side then, I started to pray about the birth and think in a more focused way about labour. As you probably know, an essential part of training for today's athletes entails their visualizing winning their event. This helps them think through in detail what they will need to do mentally in order to win – they rehearse in their mind what winning feels like. I think much can be achieved with this sort of visualization, so I tried to spend time thinking prayerfully and creatively about the sort of birth I wanted. I visualized what it would be like to feel elated, holding my baby once it was all over.

I found writing in my journal an incredibly useful exercise as I did this. I drew messy spider diagrams, noting down ways in which I planned to deal with labour pain, relaxation techniques and key Bible verses I would meditate on. Two verses I would cling on to in the toughest moments were: 1 John 4:18: 'Perfect love drives out fear', and Philippians 4:13: 'I can do everything through him [Christ] who gives me strength.' When Will and I climbed Kota Kinabalu (Asia's highest mountain) a few years back, these were the verses I meditated on, repeating them over and over in my mind throughout the climb. I used this technique during my labour too. It seems that having a baby and climbing a mountain are not dissimilar experiences: both certainly require huge amounts of endurance.

Not long before my due date, a friend at church announced to me that one of the church customs was for the whole church to be with me when I went into labour. The thought of it nearly sent me into labour then and there – when she saw my nervous expression she rapidly explained that she meant they would not be planning to come to hospital with me, but would be supporting me in prayer! One way in which this is expressed in our church community is for the women to hold a 'prayer shower' for mothers-to-be. This is like a baby shower, but instead of receiving gifts (those were given with humbling generosity post-birth), I was given something much more meaningful – a time of prayer for the birth and the health of our baby, and of prophecy for our new family. I walked away from that special afternoon with a fresh, peaceful sense that, whatever happened, whenever my baby chose to arrive, God was in charge.

Like 75% of first babies, Skye arrived late. I had expected that, as the days passed after my due date, I would become increasingly stressed. I feel massively indebted to those who were praying for me because I'm sure they were asking God to keep me calm – I really did feel surprisingly relaxed. (Of course this may have had something to do with the fact that I was at my parents' home, in a happy post-Christmas stupor of cheesy family movies, relaxing country walks and bottomless tins of Quality Street.)

I sensed my labour might be getting going following an

appointment with an aromatherapist (who was a Christian and an ex-midwife), which I had five days after Christmas. I had a 'show' as soon as I got home, and pain reminiscent of light period cramps came on. Thinking this wasn't enough to be concerned by yet, I went to bed as usual. I woke at 1am, unable to sleep further because of the pain. I felt a wave of relief that the long wait was almost over. I was also excited and nervous: what would the next level of pain be like?

Although I had arranged to send a text to one of our church friends once I went into labour – she would kick off a chain of texts asking others to pray for us – events from that point on rolled too fast for me to get round to it. My memories of the following few hours are a blurry mix of jumping in and out of baths, frantic prayers for strength, and Will giving regular reports on how far apart my contractions were.

Our journey to hospital was like a mad, high-speed car chase. The midwife we had spoken to on the phone around 4am advised us not to leave home for a good while – although we had told her we were at least forty-five minutes away. My contractions rapidly gathered pace, and by the time Will bundled me into the car, they were coming every two minutes (we were advised to be in hospital by the time they were five minutes apart). We both began to panic – giving birth on the hard shoulder of the M4 was definitely not part of our birth plan! As we drove, I tried to force myself to listen to the cheesy love songs pumping out of Heart FM in a bid to be distracted from reality – but my whole being was taken up with dealing with each wave of pain. Friends have asked how I felt at this stage, but it's a question I struggle to answer because, at that point, it seemed as if all I could manage was survival: even feelings were on hold.

Skye was born at 7.20am, two and a half hours after we

arrived at the hospital. I had wanted a water birth but this wasn't possible due to the speed with which she arrived. My disappointment about this was negated by my delight – and surprise – that I had managed the birth without pain relief, bar gas and air. I am hugely grateful to Will (my fantastic birthing partner) who largely made this possible. During our time in hospital, he took responsibility for all the decisions, coaching and encouraging me through the birth.

Although I am writing this only four months after giving birth, I already find it difficult to recall many of the precise details of the event. People say that women do forget giving birth, as does John 16:21: 'A woman giving birth to a child has pain because her time has come; but when her baby is born she forgets the anguish because of her joy that a child is born into the world.' In my experience, this verse rings true. But the memory of having a tiny little person placed on me for the first time – our tiny person, a gorgeous girl, perfectly created and fresh into the world – will never fade. That moment made every bit of pain and effort worth it.

Reflecting back on Skye's birthday, I feel the experience was essentially a positive one. God was so faithful in giving me a quick birth – one of my pre-labour prayer requests to friends had been for a labour of eight hours or fewer. (My mother had a very long labour with my brother, her first baby, and I really didn't like that idea. I'm not sure why I picked eight hours; I just felt that I have the sort of pain threshold that couldn't endure intense pain for much longer than that.) The time from when the pain started in earnest to the delivery was seven hours and twenty minutes exactly. I know that when I will look back on Skye's birth in years to come, that answer to prayer will always act as an undeniable reminder that God's presence was with us so powerfully that day.

## Catherine's birth story: Joshua

'I assumed that giving birth to Joshua was going to be a similar experience to having my first child, Sophia. She was born late, at forty-two weeks, and I actually wanted the same thing to happen the second time around. I had decided that between forty and forty-two weeks I'd do everything I needed to before the baby came. But things didn't go according to plan.

'One day in my fortieth week, my mum announced that I wasn't to have the baby as she was visiting my granny who was sick. I told her that I was actually feeling a few slight twinges of pain. I was going to a friend's house for lunch with Sophia, and, as I left to get on the bus, I joked with my husband Johannes that I'd let him know if it was a boy or a girl.

'The twinges soon became more regular but, as I wasn't yet forty-two weeks, I assumed it was nothing. When the pain increased at lunchtime, I called Johannes. He came to collect me and from there it all happened really fast. My waters broke in the car but I still wondered if this was the real thing. I was in denial that the baby was coming, perhaps because I didn't feel ready for it. I wanted to pray more; I wanted things to be more in order.

'Johannes wanted to take me straight to hospital, but I assured him we had plenty of time, so he went to drop Sophia off with a friend. Alone in the house, I began to feel really overwhelmed. Sophia's birth had been a smooth one, although she was born with a streptococcal infection. This bacterium is carried by a mother and can be passed to a baby in the birth canal. I had been told by medical staff to ensure that, with any subsequent births, I would be given antibiotics intravenously during my labour in order to prevent the baby becoming infected. Suddenly, I realized that right now I was meant to be in hospital taking the medication, and instead I was at home by myself.

'In that moment I felt really aware of how I had no control over my situation. It was one of those rare life experiences when you recognize God's greatness instantaneously. I told God, "I'm scared. I'm scared. I don't want to lose my baby." I felt genuine fear, and in that moment I had no faith. But then God spoke some words to me. He said, "Blessèd be the name of the Lord." I know they were his words because I don't express myself like that. I don't know why he spoke those particular words – they didn't make the fear go away – but I did feel then that God was with me. In the height of labour those words were at the forefront of my mind.

'When Johannes returned (he remembers that this was seventeen minutes later exactly), I could feel the baby and knew he was ready to be born. Johannes and a neighbour helped me to the car. I can see now how God was with me, even in this. We live on a really busy road but on that particular day it had been shut off, meaning that, unusually, we could park outside our house. Had that not happened and had there been a delay, doctors told us that Joshua would have been born in the car.

'In the hospital waiting room a ten-year-old boy turned to me and said, "Don't be frightened. My mum's in there and they look after you really well." I know it sounds twee, but I saw God in those small things.

'When the midwife checked me, she said the baby was ready to be born and I should push. Half of me was in delirium and I thought, "Baby, you're not meant to be here yet. Please can I have more time?" The other half of me became incredibly chilled out. I just couldn't deal with the pain. I said to God, "I can't deal with this, God. You deal with it."

'The midwife said she thought it was probably too late for the antibiotics to work, but she would give them to me anyway. Then we discovered that Joshua's head was stuck, which meant that there was more time for the antibiotics to work. It was too late for the epidural I wanted, but I was given gas and air.

'As the gas and air began to take effect, I stopped worrying. I didn't even feel any pain in the last twenty minutes of the birth. I just focused on those words that God had given me and I started to feel amazing. Some celebrities say giving birth is a spiritual experience – I would have laughed at that before, but now I can identify with it. I could hear the voices of the people in the room but I felt like I was looking down on myself. Gas and air had had no effect on me during Sophia's birth, but this time it was totally different.

'When Joshua came out I was overwhelmed – not just by seeing this new life, but also by the fact that there was nothing wrong with him. He didn't develop a streptococcal infection. After my experience of Sophia being ill when she was born, I was so nervous that he wouldn't be OK. I was thankful that he was fine and I felt elated that the birth had been so quick. I hadn't planned it like that, but I know God had been present throughout.'

## Ali's birth story: Josiah

'After having my first child, Gracie, I suffered a miscarriage. Finding out about this was very upsetting, especially as the news wasn't broken to me gently. The radiographer scanning me simply told me that I had miscarried and there was nothing to see on the scan, and then she left the room to make a phone call.

'A couple of months later, I became pregnant again, but at an early five-week scan I was told that the pregnancy had again failed. I didn't feel too surprised as it was so soon after the miscarriage. It was, however, a difficult season, as my husband Nick and I had felt that it was the right time to have a second child.

'I then had a minor operation to clear my womb. It was done by a friend who is a top gynaecologist and a Christian. Somehow he seemed to bring God's grace, some hope for the future and even some humour into our situation, as well as incredibly generously waiving his fees. Around that time, one of the leaders of our church had been talking about Psalm 84:

> Blessed are those whose strength is in you,
>      who have set their hearts on pilgrimage.
> As they pass through the Valley of Baca,[1]
>      they make it a place of springs;
>      the autumn rains also cover it with pools.
> They go from strength to strength,
>      till each appears before God in Zion.
> (Psalm 84:5–7)

Just before I went in for the operation I was praying, and I'd had those verses on my mind. When I got home after the operation, I read my Bible notes for the day, and they were the very same verses.

'During those few months my Christian friends and family surrounded me and prayed for me, and I had loads of text messages and phone calls. An amazing array of people supported me, which was really special.

'A few weeks after the operation, I still wasn't feeling right physically, and things were really uncomfortable in my stomach. I thought I had better go back to the obstetrician. He said we should do another scan as there might be something wrong. I lay down and he began scanning me. A few

moments later he said, "Well, he's waving at you." I'm glad
I was lying down, as I think it was about the most surprising
thing that anyone could have said!

'It turned out that I was eleven weeks pregnant – I had
miscarried a twin a few weeks earlier, but at the five-week
scan the doctor hadn't been able to see that there was a
second baby present. I found it incredible that my body
could deal with that happening – on the one hand bleeding
from the miscarriage, but on the other hand carrying a baby.
It was a confusing time though, a real roller coaster. I kept
wondering whether the bleeding would affect the other baby
that was there. I had also discovered this well into the pregnancy. Over Christmas I had drunk champagne and eaten
rare steak and seafood and done all the things you are not
meant to do. The obstetrician said, "Good for you!" when I
told him, which went some way to reassuring me.

'When I went for my next scan, I was told that there was
something wrong with the baby's bladder, so I had to book
in for another scan. I prayed, "Please, God, let this be fine;
let this just be nothing." And that day I wrote in my diary,
"God, would you be my shield and protector? Guard my
mind and my heart and my body with your peace." When I
returned for the scan, nothing showed up. Apparently previously there had been something wrong with the scanning
machine.

'Six weeks before my due date, my husband went away for
the weekend with our church. I went to stay with my parents
so that they could help me with Gracie, who was then three
years old. When I woke up on the Saturday morning, the
bed was soaking wet. For a split second I wondered what on
earth had happened, and then I realized that my waters had
broken. I rang the local hospital – not the hospital where I
was meant to be giving birth – and they said to come straight

in. I didn't have my hospital notes with me and, to the nurses' frustration, I didn't even know my blood type.

'Someone rang my husband, and various friends gave him lifts across the country to the hospital. Meanwhile the doctors told me that my waters had broken but the baby would be OK. I was to stay in hospital so that they could keep an eye on me over the next couple of weeks.

'An hour or so later they discovered that the baby was in a breech position and wouldn't be able to turn around to birth position as my waters had gone. Now I would need a Caesarean section in two days' time. I thought: "This isn't great, but we'll pray for the baby to turn around, so that I can give birth naturally." Friends started praying for that to happen.

'That night, I was given steroid injections to help develop the baby's lungs, which are often underdeveloped in a premature baby. I was also strapped to a machine to monitor the baby, and during the night the beepers went off. It was an emergency situation, and suddenly there were several nurses and doctors in the room all looking down at me. The baby's heart rate was dropping, and the doctors thought that the umbilical cord might be tied around him. I would need the Caesarean straightaway. They told me to phone Nick.

'Amazingly I felt completely peaceful during all of this. It was almost as if I was watching it go on, and I felt safe and surrounded by God. The only time I did feel really stressed was when I tried to ring home. Nick was staying with my parents, and all their mobiles were switched off. After a couple of long minutes I did get hold of him, and my dad brought him into the hospital just as the operation was about to start.

'I had an emergency Caesarean, which was very quick, and Josiah was born at 4 lb 9 oz. The nurses showed him to us, and then he was taken to the neonatal unit to help him breathe because his lungs were underdeveloped.

'Just after Josiah was born, Nick overheard one nurse saying to the other, "Have you seen this condition before?", and the other replied, "No, I haven't." It turned out that Josiah had a rare condition called velamentous insertion, which means that his umbilical cord was only attached very loosely to the placenta. If the pregnancy had gone full term and I had gone through natural labour, the compromised umbilical cord could easily have broken away. This is clearly very dangerous for a baby, and can result in brain damage or death. It's something that is easily missed during a scan, and the only safe method of delivery for mum and baby is by Caesarean.

'My waters breaking, and having an emergency Caesarean section, were nothing to do with that condition whatsoever, but because of those things Josiah was delivered safely. When I found out about his condition and realized how differently things could have turned out, I really felt that God had been in control all the way through. I felt a flood of thankfulness and relief.

'We were told that we might have to stay in hospital for the next month or two. But many people were praying for Josiah, and he started breastfeeding really quickly. Within three days he was putting on weight and, amazingly, we were allowed to go home. It was scary having such a tiny baby at home for the first few days, but he started to thrive straightaway.

'I was hoping to have a straightforward and wonderful water birth with Josiah, as I did with my daughter Gracie. But in a way, I am pleased I have experienced both extremes! When you give birth naturally you feel like you have climbed a mountain or run a marathon, or achieved something absolutely awesome. There is a real high after the birth. But when you have a Caesarean you can feel a bit cheated that you haven't gone through labour – I didn't have the same sense of achievement as after giving birth to Gracie naturally. But with the Caesarean Josiah was born quickly and – most importantly – safely and, as an extra bonus, there was no pain involved for me, although the recovery period took longer.

'Josiah has just celebrated his second birthday and is well into his "terrible twos" now! He is full of life and joy and mischief – and I am utterly grateful to God that he had his hand on this little boy from the very start. Psalm 139 says, "You knit me together in my mother's womb", and I have the most incredible experience of God doing just that with Josiah.'

## Your birth story

Are you wondering what birth story you will soon be telling? Each of these stories in its own way reminds me that, however much we want to plan our experience of giving birth, this is an event dictated by nature that we can't control. I was reminded of this recently by an article in the *Sunday Telegraph* under the headline: 'No such thing as perfect birth'. It highlighted the views of Sheila Kitzinger, author of twenty-five books on childbirth and parenting, speaking in response to the UK government pledge that, by the end of 2009, every woman should be able to choose where and how to give birth. While in favour of this policy, she pointed out the danger of a consumerist approach to childbirth, saying that today many women, accustomed to taking control of their careers, make the error of thinking in the same way about childbirth. Kitzinger said, 'There is a heavy emphasis on performance and achievement today. Women increasingly think that they should keep control of childbirth, rather than surrender to the experience.'[2]

Of course we do need to prepare as best we can for childbirth, but then we need to ask God to help us remain open-minded and hold his hand tightly in faith.

Prayer really can be at the heart of the birth experience, as I hope these stories have impressed upon you. God can and will intervene in the process, protecting you, your husband and your child, giving you strength to endure, and hope in him that the time of waiting for your new arrival will very soon be over. Have you invited him to take the lead part in your birth story?

## For reflection or discussion

1. Your hospital or doctor has probably encouraged you to make a birth plan. To what extent do you expect to follow this in reality? How will you feel if your birth does not match up to the plans you have made?
2. How do you hope to cope with labour on a personal level? Take some time to ask God about this and give him any fears you feel about giving birth.
3. Write down some Bible verses to keep to hand for when you are in labour, and ask some Christian friends if they will commit to praying for you when it is time for you to give birth.

## 7. THE HAND-HOLDER: DAD AND THE BIRTH

**By Will**

Louie and I have found that every book we've read on pregnancy devotes relatively little content to the father's role in the birth of his child. And few of the birth stories in books and magazines are told from a father's (or birthing partner's) perspective. But when Louie and I reflect on the day Skye was born, we realize how different our experiences seem, and that each of us has a unique story to share in terms of our interactions with God that day.

Some people journey through pregnancy alone, and will not have the father of their child present at the birth. Or it may be that, as a couple, you decide to have someone other than the baby's father take on the role of birthing partner. However, as we are focusing on the process of becoming parents as a couple in this book, we decided it would be exciting to give the subject of dads and the birth the airtime we feel it deserves. It is our hope that, whatever your own plans for the birth, you will find the accounts shared in this chapter insightful and useful to whoever plays the part of birthing partner on the big day.

Assisting at the birth of a child is a huge responsibility. It puts you face to face with pain, blood, hospitals, and many other things we generally try to avoid. At the same time, standing with your spouse in her time of need, dealing with the practical logistics of the birth and being present to hold your baby at the end of it all, are some of life's greatest privileges. During Skye's birth I prayed like never before, and the sheer wonder of seeing God's creative presence in the birth of a child is something I will never forget.

This chapter takes a similar format to Chapter 6. My own account of Skye's birth is followed by two further birth stories that other Christian fathers have shared with me.

## Will: dad to Skye

I was in a bit of a grump for the few days before Skye was born. Christmas had gone really well at church but my energy levels were depleted. I was in an emotional place that I call being 'peopled out'. So I retreated into my man-cave, which consisted of me wandering around the fields near my in-laws' home for a couple of hours each day. I knew the birth of our baby was imminent because Louie was almost a week overdue, but I didn't have the energy to get really keyed up about it all. Instead I prayed and walked, asking God for strength and protection for all of us.

On the day that Louie went into labour, she seemed to be blossoming. I did notice that she was also tired, but nothing warned me that this was the big day. She headed off for some pampering treatment that involved having smelly oils rubbed into your skin. My mother-in-law seemed to think this could make all the difference, but I was highly sceptical.

At 1am Louie jabbed me in the ribs with a moan and

the words, 'Something's happening!' I jumped out of bed and considered my next move, which was to get some paracetamol and then jump back into the bed, out of the freezing cold. Checking my watch, I felt safe in the knowledge that contractions were around seven minutes apart. I laid hands on Louie's tummy, and prayed that God would protect her and the baby through everything that was to follow.

The next few hours passed as a bit of a sleepy haze between mild contractions and me checking the second hand on my watch. At around 4am Louie jumped up, and I could tell that the pain was becoming much stronger. I got out the TENS machine,[1] although we didn't get around to using it until much later. Then I called the hospital.

It was disconcerting to be told by a midwife, 'Try putting her in a warm bath and if the contractions fade, don't bother coming into hospital for a while.' I helped Louie into the warm water at 4.15 am – an odd time to be having a bath – and she immediately yelped in pain as a massive contraction rocked her body. My man anger erupted. 'Stupid idea!' I stormed. A few minutes later we were strapped into the car and driving to the hospital in London.

I noticed that Louie's contractions had moved from being every six minutes to taking place twice within a song being played on the radio. My foot fell to the metal. We had a forty-five-minute drive ahead of us, and my initial calm had given way to a mixture of anxiety and focused speed camera avoidance.

On arrival at the hospital, I rushed Louie through into the lift. There were two buttons I could have pressed: the active birth centre where you roll around on balls (probably with a lavender infusion to ease the pain) or the medical birth suite. I knew Louie had hoped to press button one, but taking a look at her and the way things were progressing, I hit button two and hoped she would forgive me later.

Literally screaming for a doctor, we were seated on the receptionist's stool and told to wait for a room. I was battling to contain my frustration and remain polite and courteous. When we were finally shown into a room, I remember the doctor saying something about Louie being 'almost fully dilated'. This meant that the 'pushing stage' was fairly imminent.

The last thing you need on arrival at a hotel is to unpack and then get told you are going to be moved to a different room. If it's bad news in a hotel, imagine what it is like when you have a baby pushing its way out. I can't say I dealt with this demand with particular grace but, having been assured that we were now in the correct room (completely identical to the last), I focused on supporting Louie through the pain.

My mental plan was straightforward. Having spent years in rowing teams, I understood the value of staggered training rewards. I would offer different pain relief options to Louie as a reward for her time spent labouring – this way I could pace us through the long hours of labour ahead. I started by gradually increasing the zaps on the TENS machine, then would come the gas and air, and then I would suggest pethidine, and so on. As every contraction came I held Louie's hand and coached her through the pain, counting down the contraction to its fade point. It might sound like a bit of a robust approach, but knowing Louie's determined mentality, and having coached her in a rowing team, I was sure it would be the most helpful way through.

I was deeply upset at seeing Louie in so much pain during her labour. There is something very mixed about both wanting to take the pain away, and knowing that the pain also needs to increase before you see the baby. I knew I had to hold it together and be strong for Louie, but the only way I could do this was to pray for God to help her, while remaining calm and confident in the things I said. There were moments though – especially when I was alone with her – when I felt like crying and apologizing for the whole thing.

Given the intensity of the experience, I was amazed by the relaxed midwives who meandered in every so often, and having had a peek, just kept repeating, 'The baby she is a-comin'; that baby she is a-comin'' as if nothing much of any significance was actually happening. After two hours of real bed labour, a greyish walnut appeared at the business end. The midwife shouted that she could see the head and I just remember thinking, 'Oh my goodness, that is the smallest baby I have ever seen. We are giving birth to Tom Thumb!' Fortunately, but unknown to me, this was just the skin of the crown pushed into a lump and not an exceptionally small skull!

I urged Louie on, and within a minute or so a little head appeared, then a shoulder, and with a final flurry Skye's little body erupted into the arms of the waiting midwife. She let out a yell and then opened two very large eyes, at which point my heart seemed to connect with what I was seeing. Nothing can prepare you for that moment – it feels like all of the creative wonder of God has been condensed into a 7 lb 5 oz baby. I just kept staring at her on the little white towel, thinking, 'We have just had a baby. Look, that's our baby!'

### Giles: dad to Skylar

'My wife Dill had a dream in the early hours of the morning on the day of Skylar's birth. She saw herself in a tiny boat on the sea, and behind her, on the horizon, an enormous tidal wave was approaching. She felt terrified, but as she watched, instead of tossing the boat over, the wave picked the boat up and surfed her safely on to the shore. Dill told me that she felt God was showing her that the birth would be scary, but to trust him every step of the way. After what happened later, I was so pleased that God had given her that assurance. Without it, the whole experience would have been a lot more frightening.

'Contractions had started at around 10am and, because our first child, Arran (now five), had been born really quickly, I decided that we couldn't take any chances. We drove the hour from our home in the Scottish Highlands to Aberdeen Hospital. Having moved up from London only a couple of months previously, it was even more important that Dill felt settled and relaxed about it all.

'As the midwives checked Dill out, I got everything sorted for a long wait in the hospital – including my laptop, which was loaded up with *Gladiator*. But the midwives said, "No, it's not coming now; it's going to be a while yet. You should go back home and wait there until contractions develop further." So we drove the hour back home. Dill had two more episodes of this false labour on the next two mornings. But by the third day she was exhausted. In the early afternoon, she started to complain that the contractions were getting much stronger.

'I wanted to pop out and pick up our son who was at nursery, but she wouldn't be left alone, and insisted on coming along with me. As soon as we got to the nursery the contractions started again and became quite painful and so we stopped at the cottage hospital in Aboyne just to get her checked again. There was one nurse there, and she was ready to close for the evening – it was just a tiny Highland cottage hospital after all. The contractions were every seven minutes. She reassured us that it was still early on and the contractions might well fade away as before. But once we had almost reached home (heading another half-hour away from the hospital!), Dill just knew it was more urgent, and said we needed to go to Aberdeen Hospital straightaway. We did a roadside pit stop at a friend's house en route to drop off Arran, and then it was straight on to the hospital.

'Halfway through the journey, Dill started telling me she was feeling the urge to push, which was a bit worrying to say the least. I had been driving quite slowly until this point, trying to give her a smooth ride. I had driven Dill to the hospital in London for Arran's birth in my old Jeep Cherokee and she had hated the bumps in the road, so I had been trying to be more careful this time. I was thinking, "Oh no, I *still* have a half-hour drive ahead of me and Dill's talking about starting to push!" That was when I turned up the revs and really start motoring. I remember we came to one little village and it was close to rush hour. There were traffic lights ahead and the road had a queue of about twenty cars backed up. I could see that ahead there were still cars going through the lights, and so I just floored it through past all the waiting cars, at about 90 mph. They were all hooting at me. It was completely mad.

'In the countryside approaching Aberdeen there was solid traffic on a dual carriageway with no hard shoulder. Dill was screaming and started sort of standing up in the car against the passenger seat. I called the hospital on my mobile and said, "My wife is having a baby. What should I do?" In the background Dill screamed over my shoulder, "I'm not just having a baby in a month or two – it's coming right now!" She was standing up in the seat again, and at this point actually holding the baby's head in her hand. She was saying to me, "Just pull over." But I was thinking, "If I pull over, what then? What do I do then?" We had the women in the hospital shouting over the phone, "What's going on? What's happening?" And I was like, "Yes, yes, well, she is actually having the baby right now!" At the same time as all this, I was still driving in the traffic with my hand just flat down on the horn, trying to clear the cars out of the way. The drivers were obviously really angry, but I just drove up behind them, wheels spinning and honking my horn. Then they saw Dill so they let us past. It was chaos.

'I spotted an ambulance about 400 metres ahead of the traffic, so I thought, "Right, I am going to make it to that ambulance." I was honking my horn, and hitting wing mirrors as I sped past the other cars. Dill was still screaming, and the woman on the phone from the hospital was wondering what on earth was going on, but I just had to get there! I finally made it to the ambulance, but the driver wouldn't be flagged down, so I had to physically pull in front of him to stop him. I got out and ran to his window. He was indignant and said, "You know, we have got someone in the back of this ambulance." I said, "I don't care. My wife is having a baby in the car."

'The driver was only about twenty-five and looked like he had just passed his ambulance exams. I was sure he had never delivered a baby before. But he bravely knelt there by the foot well of the car, in the middle of the traffic jam on a country motorway with traffic whizzing past us. I was sitting in the driving seat supporting Dill when the baby literally just came out on to the passenger seat.

'We were shocked, and I remember saying, "Er, what do we do now? How are we going to cut the umbilical cord?" Then all these policemen turned up just like there had been a bank robbery. There were probably three squad cars and a couple of motorbikes, and they were all ready to deal with the situation. They all thought it was absolutely awesome, and as the new dad they kept coming over to me and saying,

"Congratulations, well done!" and patting me on the back. Fortunately the baby was fine.

'Another ambulance arrived and we got in the back. We were driven to Aberdeen Hospital with an incredible police escort, and motorbike outriders at the front stopping the traffic for us. A policeman kindly followed us in my car. I was thinking, "I knew I should have got the leather interior!"

'It was a surreal and traumatic experience, but there was no time really to engage with it until afterwards. Actually it wasn't until we were in hospital, and then over the following weeks, that we really got to stop and think it all through carefully. Everyone loves telling the story, and it was all over the local newspaper, but we really needed to pray it through and explore it with God.

'There was a kind of numbness about it for us, and we really had to ask God for healing, praying through the memories of the experience and praising God for his protection. Skylar was 7 lb 2 oz in the end, and perfectly healthy. Dill had done amazingly, with no pain relief, and little assistance from anyone. Looking back on it, we felt that God had been overpoweringly present. Anything could have happened, but we were never overtaken by terror. God had been with us, totally enshrouding us with his love. Obviously we were given a lot of advice that wasn't right, but God overruled and protected us and Skylar through it all. It was just like Dill's dream in the end – scary and traumatic, but God was faithful and trustworthy.'

### Benedict: dad to Charlie

'I know it sounds strange, but I was more apprehensive about how the labour would affect my body than my wife's. I have a rare arthritic condition that means I can't stand still for a long time without getting really sore. I was worried that

I might not be able to be a good support to my wife, Sam, particularly if it was a really long labour.

'On the night when Sam's labour began we had been receiving prayer ministry at our old vicar's house. People had been praying for the baby to come soon, and that night our prayers were really answered! We were in bed around 11pm when Sam said, "Some water has come out." There wasn't a lot of water, but I called the hospital anyway, and drove Sam there. In the car on the way, we were praying for wisdom about what to do. We weren't really sure whether the waters had broken fully, but we thought it was worth getting checked anyway.

'It was mid-August and absolutely roasting hot outside, so I just went in a T-shirt. It turned out that we were in the new air-conditioned prenatal suite and it was freezing. By 3am the hospital staff were quite sure Sam was not going to give birth any time soon, and so, to avoid me getting frostbite, they sent me home for the night.

'I got up early the next morning and started ringing up friends to update them on the labour and asking them to pray for us both. Because of visiting hours, I couldn't actually go back into hospital – which was a bit of a shocker for an expectant dad.

'That morning some tests had been done on Sam to check the size of the baby. The computer's results indicated that the baby was under 5 lb, meaning that when it was born it would need to be taken straight to the special care baby unit. This worrying news really upset Sam, but at the same time the midwives told her that the baby was going to be a good weight. I felt really frustrated that I hadn't been there when they had talked to Sam about this. In the end it turned out that the midwives were right and the computers were wrong!

'When I arrived back in the hospital at lunchtime, Sam was still in the prenatal ward on the top floor. This kept the delivery suite, two floors below, free for women who were in the final stages of labour. Sam's contractions were still twenty minutes apart, so we went for a walk to get a coffee and stave off her boredom. Sam actually works as a physiotherapist in the hospital, so we saw some of her colleagues, which was slightly surreal. Most of them coped with this, but when she had a big contraction some of the young male physiotherapists looked a bit awkward.

'The increasingly powerful contractions prompted us to head back up to the ward. On arrival, her dinner turned up, which she couldn't eat, but which I enjoyed. You forget how hungry you get standing around for hours on end. Sam's inability to eat, and the shortening time between contractions, definitely pointed to something happening, and so I went to get the midwife. "Just relax. Don't worry. There is plenty of time," she said.

'Sam had a shower, but that didn't help. She was sure that the baby was on the way now, so I helped her back on to the bed. I tried to tell the midwife that the baby was coming, but again she didn't believe us and wouldn't come into the room. By 9.30 pm Sam was screaming loudly in-between sucking on gas and air. I went out and said, "Look, my wife is having this baby. Come in NOW!"

'When she came in, the midwife said to Sam, "I will have a look, but when I do, I want you to calm down and have some more gas and air." It seemed she was saying that Sam was making a fuss about nothing. The midwife very casually had a look and then went pale and screamed at Sam not to push any more because she could see the head. She ran out of the door to get help.

'I felt we kept getting abandoned, and I wasn't happy at

being left alone again. I was attempting to calm Sam down and deal with the fact that the baby was about to be born, but trying to stop a woman from pushing when she is at that stage of labour is pretty impossible. I just kept offering her gas and air and hoping that the staff would be there in a minute.

'When they did come back, they pulled the bed out to move Sam to the delivery suite, but they had left everything plugged in, so we came to an abrupt stop. I went round and ripped all the plugs out of their sockets so we could actually roll down the corridor to the lift. Sam had her arms above her head and as we flew down the corridor, two doors swung back and caught both her elbows.

'We finally reached the lift and the midwife ran off down the stairs, leaving us with a couple of junior nurses. We probably waited for the lift for only twenty seconds, but it felt like an age. I was thinking, "This isn't really the best time for us to be waiting for a lift." Of course when it did arrive, I suddenly felt nervous that it would get stuck. During that journey down two floors I was probably the most anxious I had been throughout the whole labour.

'We were rushed into the first room available in the delivery suite, but there was no time to transfer Sam on to the bed. There were six staff in the room; some sorting the equipment and some looking after Sam. Thirty seconds after getting through the door, the baby was born.

'Having waited in hospital for twenty-four hours, we ended up being rushed into a room with just seconds to spare. I didn't have any time to engage with my frustration at the situation, but I distinctly remember looking at the baby, who was very quiet and purple, and thinking, "If you've killed him, I won't be best happy." We had lost twins in a previous pregnancy, so the fear of losing our next child was already in the back of my mind. I don't know what I would have done or said if that had happened. The baby didn't scream when he came out – if he had, perhaps I wouldn't have had those anxious thoughts. I wasn't overjoyed straightaway, just because I wasn't sure if he was alive or not.

'The midwives put the baby on to Sam's stomach, and he did a poo straightaway. That's when I realized everything was OK. I remember feeling quite proud of the way he had made an announcement that he was alive! It began to dawn on me that we had a little boy. I definitely wanted one of each gender, but as a dad I just remember being really proud of my little son. I cut the cord – I was really glad to do that – and gradually I began to feel more excited about it all.

'Soon everyone disappeared from the room and it was just the three of us. The happiness I felt about having a child was gradual. It wasn't like I had won the cup final – it was more of a gradual awakening. Sam went to have a shower, and I just stood there with our little baby, Charlie, in my arms. He opened his eyes and looked at me a couple of times. It was like seeing calm waters in the sea. I felt an amazing sensation of peace, like being completely chilled out. I thought, "Wow, this has finally happened." I was so happy, but I had no energy to celebrate. "Finally chuffed," was how I would describe that feeling.

'Seeing your child's birth is an awesome experience. When you see how delicate it is, it's just completely mind-blowing. The whole process of how we are made confirms to me that God exists. These are all things that I already believed, but having a child has blown my faith into a new stratosphere.'

## His story is your story

These are just three accounts of dads' experiences as birthing partners. The stories are all dramatically different but they share one great similarity: Giles, Benedict and I all tangibly felt God's presence with us at the birth of our children. The drama and the wonder of birth was wrapped up in his creative love and power. Ultimately, we recognize that we are part of his story as much as he is part of ours. Feeling the depth of our love for our children has given us a much deeper sense of God's incredible love for us.

## For reflection or discussion

1. What preparations have you made for supporting your spouse through labour?
2. Have you discussed what role you will have in the decision-making at the birth and are you fully aware of your wife's wishes regarding pain relief?
3. Have you begun to pray about the birth and have you asked others to form a prayer chain to support you when things begin?
4. What do you anticipate will be most challenging for you during the birth? Bring these things to God in prayer now.

PART IV: THE FIRST YEAR

## 8. HOW DO WE ADJUST? CHANGING
## RELATIONSHIPS AS A NEW PARENT

**By Will**

I was a little concerned when Louie recently brought home a book called *Babyshock! Your Relationship Survival Guide*. With chapter titles about rows, depression and lack of sex after childbirth, it didn't look like an easy read. The back blurb states, 'For any couple who have forgotten what it is like to be a couple because children have taken over their lives.'

In this chapter, I hope to take the shock factor out of the relational changes that occur for new parents, helping you to face them prayerfully and with excitement. If you fear being overwhelmed by parenthood, or your world already seems to have been turned on its head, don't despair. Babies have a powerful initial impact on your relational landscape, after which things transition into a new but settled pattern.

Becoming a new parent can be a final and abrupt transition from childhood to adulthood. Our thinking, outlook and expectations change and the self-interested perspectives of childhood have to be left behind. In 1 Corinthians 13:11

Paul says, 'When I was a child, I talked like a child, I thought like a child, I reasoned like a child. When I became a man, I put childish ways behind me.'

Naomi Stadlen writes, 'Having a baby – like dying – is one of the great transitions that we face, for which there can be no rehearsal. But that doesn't mean there can be no preparation. At the very least we can prepare to be disorientated and shocked.'[1] Hard as it may be, releasing the old lifestyle and expectations to God, and allowing them to die in your heart, affords you the opportunity for new life and new joy. In Matthew 16:25 Jesus says, 'For whoever wants to save his life will lose it, but whoever loses his life for me will find it.' He is teaching us that if we are willing to sacrifice our lives for him, we will find a new, wonderful life through him. Parenthood involves great sacrifice, but it offers great joy too. You cannot do Christianity half-heartedly, and in the same way you cannot successfully do half-hearted parenthood. For Louie and me, personally knowing the incredible sacrifice that God made for us so that we might be called his children, has kept the sacrifices we make for Skye in perspective.

## Your self-identity

Before we can start to rethink our relationships with others, we need to consider the effect of becoming a parent on our own sense of self. There is an unfortunate perception in our culture that having children leads to personal stagnation, rather than personal development. People with stimulating careers imagine their minds slipping into idle gear as they deal with practical chores. Parents can believe that their dreams and ambitions have to be binned as they become a mummy or daddy 'robot'. But is parenthood really like that? If we assume that life with a baby is going to mean losing all connection to who we truly are, this probably won't be a season of growth. More than that, we are likely to be a negative influence on those around us. Danny Silk says, 'Unless we learn to sustain and protect our individual health and happiness, it won't be too long before we are imparting unhealthiness and unhappiness to our children.'[2]

Becoming a mum or dad does not require dislocation from who we are or who God is calling us to be. Ephesians 2:10 reminds us, 'For we are God's workmanship, created in Christ Jesus to do good works, which God prepared in advance for us to do.' Being a parent is part of his plan for our lives, and it is often through learning to raise a family that men and women grow into new maturity and authority. Far from losing yourself, parenting can be the very making of you. Tom, dad to a six-month-old, said, 'The main way in which I've changed since becoming a parent is that I feel more of a man. Not that I didn't before, but I now feel more authoritative, stronger and more "leaderly". I also realize that lots of things that once seemed really important – like jobs, success and what people think of me – aren't half as important as they once appeared, certainly nowhere nearly as important as my daughter. This has actually meant that I'm probably better at my job, more successful, and better at relating to people because I'm less worried about how well I'm doing.'

Staying grounded in who you are means creating some healthy boundaries, and looking for the resources you need, in order to be recharged as you parent. Asking for, or perhaps paying for, the opportunity to have some time on your own can help you stay connected to yourself and God. You may consider journalling in order to help you pray about some of what you are going through. Try to embrace both the developing aspects of you as a parent, and the things that have helped to define you until now.

Time spent in God's presence is good for you, especially as you adjust to parenthood, and in the long term it's good for your baby and the other significant relationships in your life too. This is easy advice to give, but extremely hard to take, as the practical realities of being a new parent squeeze our time to the limit. However, having this intention in your mind will hopefully mean that, if an opportunity presents itself, you will seize it readily.

### Alex's story

Alex always had had a propensity to lose himself in the next new thing. He was one of those people who constantly found new hobbies or pastimes. Whatever the equipment or training, Alex would be there until he had got it mastered. Fortunately, Alex also had a wife who demanded his time, and a church leader who disciplined him to keep these hobbies in check. It was OK when it was football or cricket, but when Alex's wife Sarah became pregnant, he had a new 'legitimate' obsession.

It was as if Alex was vindicated in eating, sleeping and dreaming parenting. Rather than having it checked by his wife, she enjoyed his interest and enthusiasm, and their church leader also endorsed the new 'homemaker' Alex. The trouble was that while Alex's obsessional tendencies were being met by focusing on the baby, he was allowing an important part of what kept him balanced and healthy to die. In fact, he would have been a much better parent and spouse, had he maintained some of what he had previously enjoyed.

What had led to this imbalance was in part the sense that his leisure activities had been bad, or at least self-indulgent. The message Alex received from church had been all about self-denial and sacrifice. While it had just been the two of them in the home, he had not felt so bad about investing time in his sport. But now, with the feeding demands of a newborn imposed on his wife, he could no longer justify his own interests. So he wrote them out of the picture.

You may have heard people say, 'There's no room for self-ishness in parenting.' This is indeed true. However, there is, and there must be, space for the self in parenting. This means that your identity, which is in part reflected in your hobbies and interests, must make the journey across the bridge into your life as a parent. It may be that the scale or the frequency of these activities will need to be limited and adjusted, but they must not disappear altogether. At times – especially in the early days with a new baby – it may seem impossible to do what you enjoy, but don't let yourself believe that it is wrong to want to. God loves you as his child, parent or not, and he is happy for you to find a breadth of enjoyment and stimulation in life.

## Your relationship with your spouse

### Communication in marriage
One new dad said to us of becoming a parent, 'This is a far bigger life change than getting married.' If you are married, you will be facing this life-altering event together – making your ability to communicate arguably more important than ever before.

Every marriage book tells you that communication is the most important facet of a good relationship. Now factor in a small baby, broken nights, a full-time job, in-laws, plus a bit of colic, and you have the perfect challenge to any good communication. Natalie Williams writes in *Your Relationship Can Survive a Newborn*, 'I . . . didn't like the way that the lack of sleep and resulting frustrations changed the way Glenn and I related to each other. We had an excellent relationship and communication was central to that. Seemingly overnight this was gone.'[3]

Another reason to take the challenge of communication seriously is that, during the early months of parenthood, you will probably need to make a decision on whether mum or dad goes back to work or not, and the related issue of your new financial situation as parents. Louie and I are aware that these are big topics that we don't have the space to explore fully here. However, we do want to encourage you to consider them not only during pregnancy, but also reflect on your choices again once you are parents. Your thinking may well change: during pregnancy, Louie's plan was to return to work in the office part-time, but she has since decided to stay at home with Skye, fitting in some freelance and voluntary work around being a mum.[4] Moving from two incomes to one has been another new challenge for us, and we have needed to take time to discuss, budget and pray through these things together.[5]

There are no easy answers in resolving the challenges of a newborn to parental communication. However, be encouraged by the stories of friends who have been through it and can empathize. Remembering that this is a blip caused by a change in circumstances is essential. Retain the hope that when things settle down (and they will do), communication will recover. In the meantime ask parents or friends for help to cover you while you get some quality time together. Every little connecting point is a valuable one in the first months of being a new parent.

### Relating through sex

On average new mothers lose more than a month's sleep during the first year of their newborn's life.[6] This, combined with physical soreness, stress and breastfeeding, can mean that the intimacy 'pause button' is pressed as soon as the baby arrives. However, it is essential that the intimacy button is on 'Pause' and not on 'Stop/Eject'. Tom, one of the new parents we interviewed, said, 'We had a complicated birth, so sex for the first few months was pretty much impossible. This was frustrating, but often being too knackered meant it was less of an annoyance. I think the thing we've struggled with most is getting back into the swing of things as sex becomes more possible. The constant tiredness is a real turn-off.'

In *Who Stole Your Sex Life?* Sheila Bridge writes:

> Many, many women reported that their sex lives took second place when their children were small because they were simply too tired. Fretful toddlers pawing at you all day, combined with a baby who cries half the night, leaves anyone begging for sleep and solitude when the opportunity arises. Sex would be the last thing on the agenda.
>
> At some point after becoming a mother, it's important that you rediscover yourself as a woman and revive the interest you once felt in sex. When a short-term period of abstention becomes a long-term pattern, problems arise.[7]

Among the most challenging transitions we have seen among new parents has been this re-establishment of intimacy and romance. Hopefully some of what follows will enable you to prepare for this in advance.

One of the really important things to discuss before the baby comes is what sexual intimacy actually means to you. Why do this now? Well, the reality is that there will be a period of a month or two where sexual intimacy is not on the cards. Men in particular can find this difficult, partly because, unlike women, their hormones are still telling them that sex is a good idea. For a man, there can also be a sense of being ousted and replaced by the baby. Many find that the absence of sexual intimacy increases a sense of distance between partners. This in turn can lead to arguments, unmet needs and emotional detachment. For many men, sexual intimacy is an affirmation of love, and therefore when it is not offered they can become insecure about the relationship as a whole.

## Max and Serena's story

Max had expected a couple of weeks without sex after the birth of his first baby, and he thought he would be able to cope with that. However, after four weeks without any intimacy, Max began to make advances towards Serena, who was still exhausted and had little interest in sex. She felt that he was being selfish and unsympathetic towards her, which in turn increased his sensitivity and his desire to re-establish intimacy. Serena then became even more hostile towards Max, who was not only making unwanted demands, but was also failing to listen to her. The deadlock would be resolved only through a third party who could explain how this downward spiral had been initiated.

Talking through these sorts of realities during pregnancy can seem indulgent in the light of the fact that you are about to have a baby, but the truth is you will need to communicate effectively through this minefield.

I have always believed that regularity affords quality when it comes to sex. I am sure this is a very male perspective. Louie has always placed more value on establishing quality above frequency in our sexual relationship. Like most other couples, we struggled both with the lack of frequency and the reality that quality is often fleeting when you are exhausted, uncomfortable or interrupted by the baby! It has taken patience, trust and good communication to re-establish the intimacy we enjoyed before Skye's birth.

The best bit of advice I can give to new dads is to remember to be romantic and affirming. Many mums feel deeply insecure about their bodies after childbirth, and appreciate your compliments and attention more than ever. Make sure you keep telling your wife how beautiful and wonderful she is. She may not thank you there and then, but these things are well remembered a month down the line. Sadly many of us husbands can become ritualistic in our approach to romance, seeing it as a journey that is always headed somewhere! During this first season of parenthood, invest in it with a view to it going nowhere. Your spouse is already under a lot of new pressure, and the last thing she wants right now is a needy husband. Remember to do nice things for her: massage her aching shoulders, give her time for some pampering, make a delicious home-cooked meal. You don't need to go to town, but you do need to be a selfless romantic.

### How did having a baby affect your sex life?

'In the early stages, we felt so exhausted that the desire for sex was dramatically reduced. The bedroom became the place of one activity only: sleeping. However, as energy levels returned to nearer normality, our sex life returned also. We did have to work at it though, and it took quite some time before things returned to what they used to be.' Phil, dad to Oscar, nine months

'After the first baby, I wanted sex again long before my husband, who had problems seeing me as sexy now I was a mummy. My role had changed, and I was breastfeeding – before, my breasts had been his domain. I had to wait for him to adjust to the idea of a mother being sexually attractive. On the other hand, after the second baby, he wanted sex again almost immediately because he already saw 'mummy' as sexy and found all my nurturing very attractive. But I was so tired, I couldn't stay awake long enough.' Ruth, mum to two daughters aged four and eighteen months

'We were able to make love again about six weeks after our son arrived, but having had an episiotomy, things were rather tender. We were definitely quite tired in those early months, which did affect our love life, but obviously not too much because, after four months, we discovered we were expecting number two. We have found that pregnancy has a greater effect on our sex life because of physical restrictions and the fears of affecting the baby.' Cath, mum to Ridley, thirteen months and Bethan, one week

## Post-natal depression

As we consider how to have a healthy marriage as a new parent, I want briefly to mention post-natal depression. Worldwide, approximately 13% of new mothers suffer from PND, and if left undiagnosed it can cause significant distress to mother, child and spouse.

Confusingly, many of the symptoms of this condition are very similar to how you might feel after having a baby: sleepless, in a low mood, irritable, tearful or overwhelmed. Because of this similarity, many new mothers suffer PND in silence, unaware that they are actually unwell. Often they are overwhelmed with guilty feelings about not coping or being bad mothers. In fact the condition propagates these sorts of feelings: they are a symptom of the illness.

### Ruth's story

Ruth, mother of two young children, shared with us some of what was going on in her world when she was struggling with the onset of post-natal depression. 'Once I spent a whole day crying – in public places as well as at home – because my husband had been cross about something I had done that morning, and we had argued,' she says. 'I was sure he was going to leave me, and I would get a phone call from his best friend saying he was staying over and not coming home because I was too awful. When he returned that evening to find me still sobbing away, he had forgotten what the argument was about. He was amazed that I could think anything so ridiculous.'

Although it is not the case in every incidence of PND, part of Ruth's PND took the form of anxiety and panic attacks. She began to panic about irrational harm coming to, or even the death of, her children or husband. 'I would be afraid to go near an open window as I had mental pictures (like a flashback, but to something that had never happened) of my baby falling and being smashed on the ground. This couldn't happen because the window was too small, the baby couldn't climb, and I didn't want to throw her (I was pressed to the wall on the other side of the room), but it didn't stop the panic,' she says.

'I stopped watching films or reading because I couldn't concentrate, and the subject matter often upset me. I couldn't watch the news or read a paper as I replayed horrible stories about mothers and children in my mind, and these fed the images I had of terrible things happening to us.'

Ruth went to see her GP and was prescribed a low dose

of anti-depressants, which she took for about six months as an immediate measure. Looking back on this time in her life, she says, 'Sleep deprivation played a huge part, I think. Once I stopped breastfeeding, my elder child went to nursery and the baby started sleeping better, I felt more in control. I also tried some CBT techniques,[8] and now I feel I can push the feelings of anxiety away before they take over. My husband and I can also now recognize the signs.'

Having PND says nothing about a woman's love for her child, or her ability to be a great mother. It is a mental health condition that is very treatable and well understood. New dads can be instrumental in spotting PND, and spotting it is the key to a quick recovery. If you suspect that your wife's mood or feelings about herself or her child are significantly different from those you would anticipate in the weeks following the birth, see your GP together at the earliest opportunity. Your doctor will give her a thorough screening and, if necessary, the appropriate treatment.

## Relationships with wider family

Louie has already looked briefly (in Chapter 4) at the impact of having a baby upon your relationship with your parents. But a newborn will have an impact throughout your family, not just between you and your parents. When my sister Alice had her first son, I noticed that our relationship seemed to improve. It was like we had stopped competing with each other because she was in a completely different phase of life from me. Since then, she has gone on to have a second son, and I now have a daughter. Having children has brought us closer together, given us a new, shared story and the opportunity for a lot of fun. Somehow, it is easier to tell your sister how much you love her children, even if what you mean to say is how much you also love her.

For some people, having children can exacerbate family tensions rather than relieve them. This can be an unfortunate extra pressure for new parents. Usually, as was the case in Joseph's story,[9] a bright young child can take other family members out of the spotlight! Jealousy will rarely be directed towards your new baby, but will most likely be directed towards you. Remember that your first loyalty is to your new family, and this is not the right time to deal with wider family issues.

If things are really tough, it might be worth meeting other family members on your territory rather than on old turf. Generally most adults regress into teenage behaviour when they are all together in the traditional family home.

Some of the tensions that can arise within wider families aren't always without reason. New parents are understandably besotted with their baby and can forget sensitivities that they were previously wary of. We can also demand appreciation for our child, and be upset if that is not readily given.

Leading a church has taught me that babies can provoke some very strong feelings among adults for a broad range of reasons. If you don't feel you are getting the family reaction you hoped for, keep an open mind as to why this might be. I have counselled several people who have struggled with the arrival of a child in their wider family or circle of friends because they themselves have lost a baby, are infertile, or have had an abortion.

Just as was the case in Joseph's story, family relationships often need time, forgiveness and space to flourish.[10] But on the whole, children are a shared joy for wider families, and I expect that there are many more families that have been reunited by their arrival than have had conflicts because of them.

## Your relationship with your friends

The Bible is full of wonderful stories of great friendships, such as those of David and Jonathan; Paul and Silas; Jesus and John; and Naomi and Ruth. Most of these friendships are reinforced in times of trial and challenge. Your friendships will also be affected by the birth of your first child, and the results can be surprising. Friends are essential to your health and happiness as parents, and their ability to support and distract you in the early stages can be a real lifeline.

As a husband, I have felt a great defensiveness for Louie in this season, and have willed her friends to encourage and support her. In the vast majority of instances, we have seen incredible loyalty, love and support, not least from my church congregation who have been just fabulous. However it would be true to say that we have also felt the sting of abandonment at different times on this journey.

To a great extent, I can understand why some friendships falter. Before I became a parent, I really had no idea what it entailed: how it would affect our energy levels or opportunities to socialize. I now realize that I have probably been far less supportive than I could have been when other friends had their first children.

As a new parent, you will not, at least in the first instance, be able to invest in friendships, host events or head out to parties. It is essential that you don't feel guilty about this reality. True friends will understand, and your relationship will transcend the demands of the season. With this in mind, I suggest that you explain the realities of your situation. That way, they will at least have some opportunity to understand that life looks very different for you now.

Nothing can really prepare you for the sudden absenteeism of a trusted friend, but if you can, try to avoid seeing this as a reflection on your personality. Instead see it as a reflection of your circumstances. Trust that Jesus will surround you with many new, if unexpected, friends for this season of early parenthood, and have patience with the absent ones. They may well return when they comprehend parenthood for themselves.

## Becky's story

Becky's diary was bulging at the seams. It was worn and full of planned dates and Post-it notes with reminders of people's birthdays. Becky had always been the glue in a larger social group, the organizer, bridesmaid, godmother and party planner. She expressed her friendship as a lavish outpouring of the love of Jesus. It was her way of showing that God loved her friends and she expected nothing in return. During her pregnancy, Becky waddled around town, fitting in lots of coffees with friends, who initially laid on a lovely baby shower to see her into motherhood.

Following the birth of her son, there was an initial flurry of calls and visits, but they soon dried up. The people who did keep coming over were not the ones she had expected and, while she was glad of their company, she felt hurt that some close friends just seemed to leave her alone. Things were made worse by the stream of photos posted on a social networking site of events to which Becky had not been invited.

Becky struggled with the sense of isolation that she felt as a new parent. This was hugely exacerbated by the absence of her friends, and for several weeks she felt deeply sensitive about the matter. It was only when she joined a new mothers' support group at her church that she realized that her experience was a common one. Becky made new friends at the group and her feelings of isolation began to lift.

Aside from our wedding day, there hasn't been a single event in our lives that has led to so much contact with so many friends and family in such a short space of time as having a baby. Louie and I had forty-four visitors in the first two weeks following Skye's birth. We felt both unbelievably special and unbelievably exhausted! The intensity of all this contact, and the fact that we had a newborn in the house, was quite overwhelming. This initial flurry can also be followed by the post-celebration silence during which it is easy to feel anxious about the strength of your friendships or the intensity of your family support.

At one level, there is an inevitability about the impact of having a baby on your relationships. People will have to get used to you in your new role as mother or father. But at the same time, nothing about relationships is inevitable. Our determination to communicate well, be sensitive to others' needs, enforce boundaries and seek help will all have a bearing on how our relationships change when we become parents. The reality though for most people, including Louie and myself, was that our primary investment – indeed our sole investment relationally in those first months as new parents – was in our baby and each other. Life as a new parent has great new pressures, and this is the time to be supported, not be a supporter. If wider relationships are demanding your energy and attention, think twice about whether they are God's priority now for you as you forge the nuclear relationship of a new family.

## For reflection or discussion

1. What things might help you to process the changes you will face when you become a parent?
2. How can you improve communication with your spouse? Have you discussed your approach to intimacy during the first few months of parenthood?

3. Do you anticipate that your wider family will be supportive during this new season?
4. Which friends do you anticipate supporting you? What will you express to them about the changes ahead?

## 9. WHERE IS GOD IN ALL THIS? FAITH AS A NEW PARENT

**By Louie**

Nothing in my whole life has so disturbed and enriched my walk with God as having a baby. The following quotation from *Babyproofing Your Marriage* expresses brilliantly something of the crazy new world which I suddenly found myself in as a new parent – and which I needed to work out how to share with God:

> Meet the new boss – a tyrannical (albeit cute) despot whose demands are incessant and often indecipherable. Whatever freedom we once enjoyed is gone. If we try to make ourselves a sandwich or . . . sleep, that all-seeing, all-knowing tiny autocrat will yell his or her head off. And quite possibly take ours with it.
>
> And how about that new job description – twenty-four-hour personal servant? We all know, or quickly learn, that the work required to keep our ten-pounder alive is astounding.[1]

Having landed in the upside-down world of new parenthood, how do you hold on to – and even grow – in your faith? In this chapter I'll explore this question, using 1 Corinthians 13:13 as inspiration: 'And now these three remain: faith, hope and love. But the greatest of these is love.'

## Faith

In the first few weeks after returning home from hospital with our little bundle of joy, I recall wondering if the words 'Christian' and 'new parent' were mutually exclusive. One mother we interviewed for this book said that the best bit of pre-baby advice she was given was that those early weeks are like a black hole. Remember, you will eventually see the light, but not perhaps until you reach six or eight weeks. Another mum said, 'I have to say that in the first couple of weeks we felt like we'd been hit between the eyes with the intensity of the experience, and, of course, the tiredness.'

In the early stages of motherhood I felt so tired that praying and reading my Bible were almost impossible. Will and I bought tiny camping torches so that we could read in bed at night without waking Skye during the months when she shared our room, but I rarely made it past a couple of pages of any book before I dropped off. I began to feel as if I was drifting away from Jesus, which frustrated me. At the same time, I was too busy looking after Skye and trying to cope with life to have the time or energy to do anything about it. For the first time in years, I felt apathetic about my spiritual life.

### *Farmers and explorers*

In my experience, there are two broad approaches to Christian discipleship. There are Christians who are like Amazonian explorers, and those who are like arable farmers.

The Amazonian explorers are generally quite adaptable and are always looking for new ways of connecting with God. They often explore new models of prayer and new styles of worship with great excitement. Often the explorer type finds it hard to measure the distance travelled, such is the density of the forest. However, he or she has a permeating sense of the presence of God, regardless of how lean the times. The arable farmer, on the other hand, is very different from the explorer type. He or she enjoys established routines and follows a cycle of planting and harvesting. The arable farmer is usually aware of how things are going during the season, and can usually make close comparisons with the season before.

So what has all this got to do with parenting? Well, when your baby arrives, your discipleship style will, in part, determine how you cope with his or her impact upon your spiritual journey.

### Jess and Kelly's stories

Jess had learned the value of a daily quiet time as a teenager. She rigidly protected the half-hour that she spent reading the Bible each day, and sought a solitary place to pray alone. She had seen that this space was essential to her spiritual walk, and could look back to other seasons when this investment had produced real fruit for the kingdom. When baby Sam arrived, Jess was overjoyed, but after the initial weeks she became increasingly frustrated that her quiet time had disappeared. Having lost her protected space with God, Jess felt deep guilt at having 'abandoned' him. She began to wonder if his presence was still with her.

Jess's story is a classic illustration of the arable farmer, an approach to discipleship that presents distinctive benefits as well as some challenges. One of the great things about her story is that Jess actually missed the time she spent with God; her passion to press into him was not lost in the haze of new parenthood. Jess could recognize the difference in season, but longed to stay connected to the Lord. She would ultimately learn that the timing and the silence were less important than taking an opportunity – even if it was a less-than-ideal one – to pray and read the Bible. She ended up adapting her preferred approach to the new demands of parenthood. She read the Bible in the bath after Sam had fallen asleep. She would pray out loud while walking him around the park each day. Ultimately Jess found she could establish new spiritual routines as a parent that became part of a valuable new season in her walk with God.

Kelly had always had a more erratic approach to discipleship, but she was nonetheless a deeply prayerful and committed follower of Jesus. Her journey of faith had included a wide number of different prayer and worship styles, and she enjoyed and benefited from variations to her routine. When her daughter was born, Kelly found her prayer life invigorated – now she had a new reason to pray.

Over time, Kelly's prayer life seemed increasingly to centre on the life of her baby. She neglected her own spiritual needs, and while she was pleased that her baby was steeped in prayer, she began to feel dry and resentful. Each time she went to church, she would end up in crèche and she rarely heard any teaching. Six months later she felt like the spiritual adventure of parenthood had left her lost and hungry in the jungle.

Kelly's story is also a common one among new parents. Adventure-orientated individuals often find the spiritual transition into parenthood easier than their farming counterparts. However, their adaptability can also be a problem.

The obvious danger is that so much adaptation takes place that a new parent loses sight of his or her own relationship with God.

Equally, for adventurer types, once the initial novelty has worn off, they can feel deeply frustrated that things have become so routine. Kelly had to become resourceful and flexible in the way she re-established her spiritual journey. She bought an MP3 player and listened to a diverse array of speakers while out and about with her daughter. In church she enlisted the help of a friend so that they could swap responsibility for their babies during different parts of the service. Kelly stayed upbeat and received prayer by asking a mentor to come over once a month while her baby was having an afternoon nap.

Neither the farmer nor the adventurer is a 'better' model of discipleship. These things tend to be quite automatic, and are just a result of different learning styles and temperaments. The key question is: do you desire to be fed by God as a new parent? Flexibility and patience are needed to establish new spiritual patterns. Being resourceful and imaginative will also help you to embrace a new routine of time with God that works in your day-to-day life as a new mum or dad. Nicky, mum of two, said after she had her first baby: 'I found it hard to have formal quiet times. So I left notes everywhere in my home: inspirational quotes, and short Bible passages. As a mum you have very little reading time, but lots of thinking time.'

## Hope
While I was shocked by the sense of spiritual bleakness and apathy I felt as a new parent, there were also strange moments of incredible hope and peace. I remember praying over our tiny, brand new baby in her cot in the pitch black of

night, thanking God for her and marvelling at our Creator as
never before. I also felt a new sense of peace and 'rightness'
in my spirit about starting a family, and this was reflected
in my own relationship with my parents improving when
I myself became a parent. As Will expressed it in Chapter
8, our relationship as a couple was certainly strained at
times during the early weeks, but I also sensed that God
was bringing us into a new season which would be good
for us.

When Skye was four months old, a friend and I launched
a ministry through our church, reaching new parents in our
area. We are partnering with our local medical practice to
offer baby-weighing and health advice to new parents, with
friendship-building at the core of our ministry. We have
seen an incredible take-up for the service, and many people
are connecting with the church because of it. Where I have
stepped out in faith and served God this year – sometimes
with a sense that I have absolutely nothing to give spiritually, emotionally or physically – there has been real blessing.
Writing this book has been another ministry project that has
at times been a fantastic way to keep me focused on God and
keep my brain cells (sort of) alive. At the same time there
have been moments when I have questioned whether it was
a sensible thing to try to do at all, and I have sometimes wondered how we will ever get it finished.

I think the contrasts in my spiritual experience – from
enduring lows to incredible highs with God – reflect the
nature of early parenthood. The authors of *Babyproofing Your
Marriage* write:

> Once that baby is placed in our arms, we pass over to the other
> side. Becoming a parent is, without parallel, the single most
> beautiful moment in life . . . At the same time, new parents can

feel afraid, confused and sometimes downright miserable. How is it possible to stand there at the side of the cot . . . and feel such extreme, and diametrically opposed emotions – pure joy and sheer terror – rise within you?[2]

## *We never pray together any more*

Maintaining your joint journey of faith during early parenthood is one of the greatest challenges most couples face. It requires both parents to be present, which in itself is no mean feat with a newborn. However, if we are going to hold on to hope in God through this season, we need to share the trials and bring them to God together in prayer. Feeling isolated is also a common experience among new mothers, and praying with your spouse – or other Christians if possible – can help protect us from this.

I remember the moment when I first expressed my frustration to Will that our morning prayer and Bible-reading routine had got lost among the new busyness of starting the day with a baby in tow. As the spiritual farmer in our relationship, I found this very difficult. Things were also strange for Will (the more natural adventurer) as in the past I had often challenged him spiritually, and now I had no resources to do so. Suddenly there was a need for him to provide all the structure and motivation for our time with God. Although I was doing the majority of the night-waking, his nights were still broken for months on end. He was already leading a church, and now he also had constantly to take the lead spiritually at home.

This year we have learned to seize the moment with God. We have often found that our most lengthy spiritual conversations and prayer times happen while driving. Skye usually falls asleep in the car, and we are uninterrupted by the distractions at home. At the same time, even when we have managed to carve out shared space with God at home, the energy to do anything more than relax is often lacking. I have had to choose, in faith, to be enthusiastic about praying with Will, when my body just tells me that I should take the chance to lie down and sleep, or vegetate in front of the TV.

Developing new rhythms of time with God together has been a difficult journey for us, but despite the challenges, we are still aware of his faithful presence in our lives. We are learning many new things about him through Skye. We are softening, maturing and seeing his Spirit at work in our little child. And this season requires us to learn creativity in practising our day-to-day faith like never before. In many ways, we know that the battle to retain our joint spiritual journey is more important than the time itself. As long as we retain the passion to seek God together, he will help us to put that desire into practice in our lives.

We have been encouraged to know that we are not the only new parents battling on this front. Ian, dad to three girls under seven, said, 'I had been a Christian for almost eighteen years when our first child, Hannah, was born. In that time I had developed a routine of Bible reading and prayer that fed me spiritually before I began my day. Hannah arrived and the routine went! I was discouraged by this seemingly downward slide in my faith, until a wiser and older Christian (and father of four) encouraged me that this was quite normal in new seasons of life. What I needed, he suggested, was a new routine for a new season. Gradually I discovered other times to pray (not necessarily when I read the Bible) and I learned to walk with God more throughout the day.'

**How did your spiritual life change when you became a parent?**

'The big change is time – or relative lack thereof. I find I have to be more organized and more disciplined to get my quiet time in, and I've also had to be more flexible and just try to squeeze something in at a spontaneous moment in the day. Also, when Reuben was much younger, though we went to church, I couldn't really concentrate well, as he was often hungry or crying, making it difficult to participate.' Gayle, mum to Reuben, sixteen months

'I am increasingly aware of the need and desire to model a healthy Christian spiritual life to my children (in my relationship with Jesus, my husband and my friends), which is something that I hadn't given much thought to before.' Nicky, mum to twins Felicity and Juliette, two

'As a new mum, you can feel guilty about how busy you are, and maybe jealous that your husband can have quiet times more easily than you. I found that asking my husband to make sure we did a daily Bible study really helped. I also found that praying in the middle of the night while breastfeeding was good.' Tilly, mum to Naomi, four, and Sebastian, two

## Guilt

Novelist Fay Weldon wrote: 'Guilt is to motherhood as grapes are to wine.'[3] A sense that both my own personal faith and my shared spiritual journey with Will were in a precarious place, when God had just blessed me with the most wonderful daughter, left me feeling guilty.

Almost every book on motherhood I've picked up devotes pages to this subject. If it isn't our own spiritual life (or lack of) that we feel guilty about, we are probably feeling bad that we are not meeting our own high standards for how we raise our children. Or we are blaming ourselves for their faults as we discover that they are not 100% perfect. Again, the challenges of caring for a newborn – a task in which most mothers seem to feel deficient the first time round – can make us more susceptible to suffering from guilty feelings. One mum said, 'I found the first six weeks so hard. I felt a failure. I was incredibly emotional and found it hard to see the end of it . . .'

Stormie Omartian writes,

> When things go wrong in our children's lives, we blame ourselves. We beat ourselves up for not being perfect parents. But it's not being a perfect parent that makes the difference in a child's life, because there are no perfect parents. None of us are perfect, so how can we be perfect parents? It's being a *praying* parent that makes the difference.[4]

Stormie is right: instead of striving for perfection, we need to pray. But if you feel desperately guilty for not praying much, getting going again is no easy task.

The problem with remaining in a place of guilt is that it drives us even further from God. The worse I felt about not spending enough time with him, the less inclined I felt to give him any time I did have. Although my friend, Jenny, who recently had a baby, was fabulous in bringing her cuddly newborn to church every week, I struggled with this and so initially missed out on another point to meet with God.

## Love

> I am he, I am he who will sustain you.
> I have made you and I will carry you.
> (Isaiah 46:4a)

I love this verse, with its feminine connotations of a God who sustains and carries us, just as I physically sustained and carried Skye through pregnancy. Allowing myself to accept that this really is what God does for me has helped me turn a corner spiritually over the past few months. I have learned the hard way that my relationship with God cannot depend on my ability to draw near to him. Nor can it depend on my fervour for quiet times, or my ability to read or concentrate. I have slowly come to realize that God really does understand that at times – even for months on end – those things just aren't possible.

I want to encourage you that God is so gracious to you through the turbulence of this season. He is patient and forgiving, and his love is not dependent on what we do or don't do. Looking at the way we feel about, and respond to, our own children can teach us something fresh about his limitless love for us. Amelia, mum to Harriet, twenty-two months, said, 'One of the amazing things that happened soon after Harriet arrived was the completely overwhelming love that I started to feel for her. It was unlike any other love I have for anyone else. It threw me a bit, because I thought, "Is my love for God as strong as this?"'

Many mothers similarly report feeling a depth of love for their baby that they never knew they had within them. The incredible thing is that God loves you even more than you love your child. Sarah, mum to Arthur, six months, and now twenty-two weeks pregnant, said, 'That feeling of utter love for one's child (felt most of the time) helps us accept God's love for us. I have felt his love and grace when I haven't really had the time to spend with him this year. I just feel that he sees and understands.'

## Sacrifice

One mum of two children under four said, 'Motherhood is about sacrifice. Before I was a mum, I heard someone say this and thought they were very arrogant, but now I know better! Sometimes I get tired of the sacrifice, but you have to go on doing it or your children suffer. People often talk about mums having "let themselves go", meaning they haven't got their figure back into shape, and may well be too tired to bother ever doing anything about it. But actually, you have to do a lot of "letting yourself go" in terms of your interests, use of time and hobbies (what are they, again?). Your child takes priority, and you have to keep learning to sacrifice over and over again.'

At times I have struggled not to resent the limitations to my freedom that parenthood brings. But when I think about Skye, and how I want her to know that she is deeply loved, I want to choose to put her first. Phil, dad to Oscar, said, 'Since becoming a parent, I've had to become more selfless. In a similar way to getting married, having children highlights certain attitudes that you were unaware of. I realized I had become quite selfish, and I've been working on becoming less so ever since.'

Sacrificing my own selfish desires in order to meet Skye's needs has also taught me something new about the nature of God's love. During the past year I might have missed out on going to the cinema, washing my hair when I wanted to, or jumping on the Tube and meeting a friend at the drop of a hat. But how much more did God give when he sacrificed his own Son on the cross in order to offer me salvation? Letting go of a job I really enjoyed because of my sense that in this season God wants me to invest in my child before my work has been one of the most painful sacrifices I've made this year, and a big step of faith. As a parent, I understand the word 'sacrifice' in a new way.

### Find ways to receive God's love

When life becomes all about tirelessly giving, receiving God's love becomes paramount. We might struggle to be disciplined in quiet times as new parents, but we desperately need refuelling by his Spirit. Many of my times with God during these past months have entailed just being in his presence while walking Skye in our local park, or while quietly breastfeeding her before bed. Sometimes I have prayed, mainly telling God about the things worrying me and stressing me out. I regularly find myself praying in tongues, as it doesn't require thinking in the same way that prayer in English does.[5] I have become much more content just to be in God's presence – without the pressure of thinking about how to intercede or worship more effectively. I am sustained by these moments in my day.

Church is another way to be refreshed in your spirit. When Skye was born, we were overwhelmed by the love of our church. We were showered with cards, gifts and delicious meals. I realized, however, that the important thing wasn't simply receiving the gifts and generosity of our church community. Their actions communicated that we had brought a child into a new family who were committed to loving her, and investing in her life.

If your church runs a crèche during services, enabling you to leave your child with caring volunteers while you enjoy worship or a sermon without distractions, my advice is to make the most of it. This is something we are still developing at our church and it has meant that I have hardly heard a full sermon in the past year. I have also often found it impossible to talk to all the people I want to at church (when the baby is with you, part of your brain is constantly focused on their needs, and so I am always distracted). As a result, I can quickly feel disconnected from Christian fellowship. I do love being married to a vicar (well, this one in particular, anyway), but it does mean that you don't always have your spouse to share the baby load during a service. This has given me a tiny glimpse into the world of a single parent, and has left me in awe of how many cope so well with the challenge of parenting alone every day.

Have you connected with the other new parents in your church? If you are a parent-to-be, getting to know someone with slightly older children than yours can also be a real help – they will often be able to relate to your experience and encourage you in the early weeks. Psalm 68:6a says, 'God sets the lonely in families.' God has set you in his family, the church – let them support you and remind you of his love during a time when you really need to know it.

## Parenting as a child

In an interview with *Christianity* magazine, Sila Lee said, 'When it comes to parenting, it's as if God has put us in his place – "In loco Dei" – to our kids. Everything we model is a picture of how God loves us. It's an awesome responsibility.'[6]

Sila's words remind me that every time I serve my daughter, I am modelling his love to her. In a culture that gives little recognition to the hard and selfless work of motherhood, I need to be reminded that everything I do for my daughter teaches her what love is. When I think about the magnitude of the task ahead in raising her to know God's love for herself, I often feel overwhelmed. I need to bask in the love of God, allowing him to parent me as I learn to raise children in the light of his example.

Will recently told the over sixty-fives' group at church that they were all little children before the Lord, which I think they mainly appreciated! The reality is that whether you have a new baby or a gaggle of grandchildren, you are adopted into the Lord's family. He has no harsh expectations for your performance, and having entrusted you with a child, he will continue to parent you himself.

I believe that understanding ourselves as God's children is key to parenting. Regardless of your own familial experiences or lack thereof, God says to you, 'I am your Father. You have a condition-free position in my family.' There will be times in the early stages of parenthood when you just want to curl up in the corner and cry your eyes out. The Lord is there in those moments, as your Father, non-judgmental and full of compassion. At every step along the way, joyful or sad, ask and include him in the journey. He is your Father and he is also the Father of your new child. Nothing is too mundane or insignificant for him, and as his child, never forget to ask.

## Embrace the change

### How have you changed since becoming a parent?

'Parenthood has made me much more aware of how I behave, and my insecurities – I don't want to pass them on to my children so I try to relax more and enjoy special moments with my baby. I also trust myself to make decisions now. As a mother, you often find yourself alone with your newborn, and you can't rely on other people to help you make the right choices. I've learned to take charge of both our lives and hopefully make the best choices in bringing up my baby – I would never have asserted myself this way before motherhood.' Lydia, mum to Harry, eighteen months

'I haven't changed as much as I thought I might – I'm glad that Tom and I haven't suddenly turned super-sensible overnight! I am more tired and less organized. I have realized how much I previously sought to control everything in my life. The fact that April is entirely unpredictable and uncontrollable has brought this into stark reality. I'm engaged in a very long process of letting go.' Ellen, mum to April, six months

'I have got more in touch with my heart and emotions since the arrival of our son. Having a baby unlocks certain emotions, and enables you to access parts of your heart that you were previously unaware of.' Phil, dad to Oscar, nine months

'My lifestyle has certainly changed dramatically since becoming a parent – some of that has been easy and some more challenging. It feels like the most extreme growing up experience. Getting married was part of that process, but having a baby accelerates it to a whole new level. You are continually called to prefer somebody else, to meet their needs before your own, and to be all the things it talks about in 1 Corinthians 13: loving, kind, patient and forgiving. Many times you realize how far short you fall, so there are sometimes feelings of inadequacy. Fundamentally, as a new parent, the focus of your life shifts.' Cath, mum to Ridley, thirteen months and Bethan, one week

Brian, father of two, and grandfather of three, said to us recently, 'Becoming a parent changes everything: but I wouldn't change anything back.' Becoming a parent does change you. Yes, it changes your lifestyle, but more than that, parenthood changes your heart.

We want to leave you with a final quotation from a mum of a six-month-old: 'Becoming a parent has taught me to trust. When our daughter was really young, I can remember regularly stooping to peer over her crib, wondering how on earth I would ever be able to keep her safe, look after her properly, and be the mother she deserves. It makes me feel so helpless, but when I pray, I usually get the sense that God is saying, "Just leave her to me. Be all that you can for her. And leave the rest to me."'

For Will and me, the past eighteen months have been a time of incredible transition. The journey has been both painful and wonderful, as expressed through many of the stories in this book. Through it all, God has been unchanging, faithful, and our strength in times of weakness. The gift of Skye has been our greatest delight, and we believe you will feel the same joy when your parenting journey begins.

## For reflection or discussion

1. How might you creatively adjust your time with God to fit in with new family life?
2. Are you experiencing the love of a church family at the moment?
3. To what extent are you letting God parent you?
4. In what ways could you further receive God's love?

## APPENDIX
## PRAYERS FOR PREGNANCY, BIRTH AND
## THE EARLY DAYS

**By Will and Louie**

During pregnancy or as a new parent, it can sometimes be hard to know what to pray. In fact, it can be hard to pray at all! Since becoming parents, Louie and I have found that we have returned to using some liturgical prayers, simply because they offer words that our tired minds can't provide. We felt it might benefit you if we wrote some prayers and reflections that you could refer to at different times during your pregnancy, birth and early parenting phases. They may be all you can manage, or they may become the starting point for a longer time with the Lord. Either way, we encourage you to keep inviting God into the heart of everything that you are going through. He doesn't need your extended prayers – he just longs to be welcomed in.

### Prayer following conception
Verse for reflection: Genesis 4:1:
> 'Adam lay with his wife Eve, and she became pregnant

and gave birth to Cain. She said, "With the help of the LORD
I have brought forth a man."'

Lord Jesus,
Thank you that you have blessed us with this delicate new life.
We entrust his or her growth and development to you. Bless
us as we begin the physical, emotional and spiritual journey
towards being parents. Protect our hearts as we face the potential
hardships as well as the joys. Give us an abundance of your love
for this child as he or she grows to maturity, and make us into the
parents you want us to be. Keep us trusting you every step of the
way, so that no matter what happens in the weeks ahead, we will
know your lordship and sovereignty over us all.
Thank you for being our Creator and Protector.
In your name,
Amen

## Prayer during morning sickness
Verse for reflection: Mark 4:39:
   'He got up, rebuked the wind and said to the waves,
"Quiet! Be still!" Then the wind died down and it was com-
pletely calm.'

Lord Jesus,
You slept in a boat during a great storm, and you know the storm
that is raging in my body at this time. I thank you that, even
though I feel unwell, you are in the boat with me and have the
power to calm the waves of nausea I am experiencing.
   I don't have the energy to praise you, God, or the strength to
raise my hands, but you know that my heart is for you. I long for
you to bring me release from this sickness. I pray that you would
enable my body to adapt to the changes of pregnancy, and I
thank you for the work of preparation you are doing through

these new hormones. Protect my child, and be gentle to me in
this.
By the power of your Holy Spirit,
Amen

## Prayer before a scan
Verse for reflection: 1 Corinthians 13:12:
'Now we see but a poor reflection as in a mirror; then we
shall see face to face. Now I know in part; then I shall know
fully, even as I am fully known.'

Lord Jesus,
We feel such a heady mix of emotions as we anticipate seeing the
first scan of our baby: excitement, anxiety and nervousness. We
know that you can see far more than we will, and we trust our
child's development into your hands. We pray that we would feel
a deep connection to our baby as we look at him or her, and we
ask that you will use this event to prepare us for the face-to-face
meeting that is to come.
    Thank you for the wonder of the technology we have
available, and the medical staff serving us. Give us grace-filled
hearts towards them, regardless of the outcome of today's scan.
We know that you are sovereign over all things, and we ask you
to give us trusting hearts.
Thank you, Jesus,
Amen

## Prayer when you are worrying about your baby
Verse for reflection: John 14:27:
'Peace I leave with you; my peace I give you. I do not give
to you as the world gives. Do not let your hearts be troubled
and do not be afraid.'

Dear Lord,

Today I have been worrying about my baby. I have experienced sensations or a stillness that is making me nervous. Give me the conviction to express my concerns, and the courage to trust you. I want to be realistic and not driven by fear, but I also want to be wise and listen to my body's rhythms. Help me, Lord, by the power of your Holy Spirit, to discern what I should do at this time. Would you fill me now with deep peace in my heart so that I will know your presence with me? I need to know that I am not alone right now. Please place your loving arms around me.

In Jesus' name,

Amen

## Prayer for your marriage relationship

Verse for reflection: Isaiah 58:11:

'The LORD will guide you always;
    he will satisfy your needs in a sun-scorched land
    and will strengthen your frame.
You will be like a well-watered garden,
    like a spring whose waters never fail.'

Dear Lord,

Protect our relationship in this time of transition. Deepen our commitment to each other, and give us patience as our energies and abilities are altered by pregnancy. Steer us through the turbulence of our feelings, and give us the insight to see the truth in times of confusion.

Lord, help us to be real about our expectations for each other, but also gentle in the way we express ourselves. Would you strengthen our relationship in preparation for parenthood, so that we can be generous with our love and feel secure as we focus our attentions on our child?

In Jesus' name,

Amen

## Prayer before the birth

Verse for reflection: Joshua 1:9:

'Have I not commanded you? Be strong and courageous. Do not be terrified; do not be discouraged, for the LORD your God will be with you wherever you go.'

Dear Lord,

Give me courage to face the pain of childbirth with confidence. I know that you have built my body to be strong enough to deliver this child safely. Please minister to me through the different stages of birth. I commit myself and our child into your care now. I ask that the medical staff and midwives communicate with us well, and I trust my birth plan and pain relief to your wisdom and their hands. Give me the confidence to express my opinion, and the humility to accept advice for the well-being of my unborn child. Hem me in on every side, and fill the room with a tangible sense of your divine presence.

In Jesus' name,

Amen

## Prayer during labour

Verse for reflection: Jeremiah 33:3a:

'Call to me and I will answer you.'

Meditate on or repeat this verse:

'Be pleased, O LORD, to save me;

    O LORD, come quickly to help me.'

(Psalm 40:13)

## Prayer for when you go overdue

Verse for reflection: Psalm 37:7a:

'Be still before the LORD and wait patiently for him.'

Lord God,

I have waited for so long for this baby to arrive – and I feel I can't wait a moment longer! Help me to be patient and to relax during this time. Thank you that you have all things in your hands, including the timing of our baby's birth. I pray now for his/her health: would you watch over and protect him/her? Give the midwives and hospital staff wisdom as they decide the best step to take next in our situation.

Lord, we declare again that we believe in your awesome love and great power. Intervene in our lives: we trust in you.

In your holy name,

Amen

## Prayer for a newborn

Verse for reflection: Psalm 139:13–14:

'For you created my inmost being;
   you knit me together in my mother's womb.
I praise you because I am fearfully and wonderfully made;
   your works are wonderful,
    I know that full well.'

Praise you, Jesus! You knit this little child together in my womb. He/she is a precious gift for us, fearfully and wonderfully made in your image. We commit this child to you as a sign of our gratitude, and we pray that you would fill him/her with your Holy Sprit.

Would you help us to nurture this little baby into the man/woman that you have called him/her to be? Give us the confidence to take him/her into our home and become family there together. You have honoured us with this child, and we honour you as our Heavenly Father, who gives good things to those who love and fear him.

We bless you as you have blessed us.

In Jesus' name,

Amen

## Prayer for a new family

Verse for reflection: Isaiah 43:19a:

'See, I am doing a new thing!

Now it springs up; do you not perceive it?'

Lord God,

Thank you for the incredible new thing you are doing in our lives. We are no longer a married couple, but a family! Teach us what it means to live as a family, seeking to honour, please and serve you. Equip us to love one another as you love us – without counting the cost. Bring us joy through one another, and help us to celebrate all that you do in us and through us. May our family shine as a light for you, and bring glory to your name.

By your powerful Spirit,

Amen

## Prayer for sleep

Verse for reflection: Matthew 11:29–30:

'Take my yoke upon you and learn from me, for I am gentle and humble in heart, and you will find rest for your souls. For my yoke is easy and my burden is light.'

Dear Lord,

You grant rest to the weary and a light yoke for the burdened.

Father, I feel exhausted and challenged by the relentless demands of parenting, and I lack the sleep I need to function well. Please come close to me and restore me.

Give me grace and patience with my new baby and keep me free from frustration. I know that, despite my lack of sleep, you can and will sustain me through the small hours of the night and into the dawn. Give me courage and fortitude, knowing that while this season is hard, it will pass and rest will return once again. Minister your restoration to me, through the power of your Holy Spirit.

In Jesus' name,

Amen

## Prayer for new parents

Verse for reflection: Galatians 5:22–23:

'But the fruit of the Spirit is love, joy, peace, patience, kindness, goodness, faithfulness, gentleness and self-control.'

Father God,

Praise you for the privilege of becoming a parent! It is an awesome responsibility, and sometimes I feel overwhelmed by the lifetime calling that I have just stepped into. Thank you that you promise in your Word to give us all we need. Philippians 4:13 says, 'I can do everything through him who gives me strength.' Lord, give me the strength of character I need to raise a godly family. Help me to grow the fruit of your Spirit in my heart, and in that of my child.

Thank you that you are the first and most beautiful Parent of all. Parent me, Lord, as I learn how to parent.

In your name,

Amen.

# FURTHER READING

Most of the books below were written by Christians. We have also included some secular titles and websites that we found particularly helpful.

## On pregnancy

Jane Bullivant, *Dear Lord, I Feel Like a Whale! Knowing God's Touch Throughout Your Pregnancy – and Beyond* (Monarch, 2004).

Kaz Cooke, *The Rough Guide to Pregnancy and Birth* (Rough Guides, 2001).

Dr Anne Deans, *Your Pregnancy Bible* (Carroll & Brown, 2003).

Vicki Iovine, *The Best Friends' Guide to Pregnancy: Or Everything the Doctor Won't Tell You* (Bloomsbury, 1997).

Frances and Judith MacNutt, *Praying for Your Unborn Child* (Hodder and Stoughton, 1988).

Lindsay Melluish, *New Baby: Bible Readings for Special times* (Bible Reading Fellowship, 2006) (A month-long devotional for new parents).

## On caring for your baby in the first year

Simone Cave and Dr Caroline Fertleman, *Your Baby Week by Week: The Ultimate Guide to Caring for Your New Baby* (Vermilion, 2007).

Gary Ezzo and Robert Bucknam, *On Becoming Babywise: How to Give Your Infant the Gift of Nighttime Sleep* (Parent-Wise Solutions, Inc., 2006).

Tracy Hogg with Melinda Blau, *Secrets of the Baby Whisperer: How to Calm, Connect and Communicate with Your Baby* (Vermilion, 2001).

Rachel Waddilove, *The Baby Book: How to Enjoy Year One* (Lion Hudson, 2006).

## For new mums
Rob Parsons, *The Sixty-Minute Mother* (Hodder and Stoughton, 2000).
Naomi Stadlen, *What Mothers Do: Especially When It Looks Like Nothing* (Piatkus, 2004).
Naomi Starkey, *Good Enough Mother: God at Work in the Challenge of Parenting* (Bible Reading Fellowship, 2009).
Alie Stibbe, *Barefoot in the Kitchen: Bible Readings and Reflections for Mothers* (Bible Reading Fellowship, 2004).
Susan Alexander Yates, *And Then I Had Kids: Encouragement for Mothers of Young Children* (Baker, 2002).

## For new dads
Steve Chalke, *The Parentalk Guide to Being a Dad* (Hodder and Stoughton, 2000).
John Eldredge, *Wild at Heart: Discovering the Secret of a Man's Soul* (Nelson, 2006).
Rob Parsons, *The Sixty-Minute Father* (Hodder and Stoughton, 1997).
www.dadtalk.co.uk

## On marriage
Christopher Ash, *Married for God* (IVP, 2007).
Stacey Cockrell, Cathy O'Neill and Julia Stone, *Babyproofing Your Marriage: How to Laugh More, Argue Less and Communicate Better as Your Family Grows* (HarperCollins, 2007).
John and Stasi Eldredge, *Love & War: Funding the Marriage You've Dreamed of* (Hodder and Stoughton, 2010).
J. John, *Marriage Works* (Authentic, 2002).
Nicky and Sila Lee, *The Marriage Book* (Alpha International, 2009).

## On parenting as a Christian

Anne Atkins, *Child Rearing for Fun: Trust Your Instincts and Enjoy Your Children* (Zondervan, 2004).

Patrick Kavanaugh, *Raising Children to Adore God: Instilling a Lifelong Passion for Worship* (Chosen Books, 2003).

Nicky and Sila Lee, *The Parenting Book* (Alpha International, 2009).

Lindsay and Mark Melluish, *Family Time* (Kingsway, 1999).

Stormie Omartian, *The Power of a Praying Parent* (Kingsway, 1995).

Sue Palmer, *Toxic Childhood: How the Modern World is Damaging Our Children and What We Can Do about It* (Orion Books, 2007).

Danny Silk, *Loving Our Kids on Purpose: Making a Heart-to-heart Connection* (Destiny Image, 2008).

Care for the Family, www.careforthefamily.org.uk

John and Susan Yates and family, *Building a Home Full of Grace* (Baker, 2003).

## On parenting alone

Diane Louise Jordan, *How to Succeed as a Single Parent* (Hodder and Stoughton, 2003).

Cheer Trust, www.cheertrust.org

## On post-natal depression

Hazel Rolston, *Beyond the Edge: One Woman's Journey out of Post-natal Depression and Anxiety* (IVP, 2008).

Mind and Soul, www.mindandsoul.info

## Parenting courses

As 2 Become 3, a day-long course for pregnant couples expecting their first child, www.as2become3.org

The Family Time Parenting Children Course, see Lindsay and Mark Melluish, *Family Time: The Book of the Course* (Kingsway, 2002).

The Parenting Course – www.htb.org.uk/parenting

# NOTES

## Chapter 1

1. Elizabeth Martyn and Relate, *Babyshock! Your Relationship Survival Guide* (Vermilion, 2001), p. 34.

2. See Genesis 25:22.

3. For more on the ethics of IVF, see John Stott, John Wyatt and Roy McCloughry (ed.), *Issues Facing Christians Today*, 4th edn (Zondervan, 2006).

4. Elizabeth A. Hambrick-Stowe, *Expecting: A Christian Exploration of Pregnancy and Childbirth* (Judson Press, 1979), p. 19.

5. Naomi Stadlen, *What Mothers Do: Especially When it Looks Like Nothing* (Piatkus, 2004), p. 38.

## Chapter 2

1. Kent Nerburn, *Letters to My Son: A Father's Wisdom on Manhood, Life and Love* (New World Library, 1999).

2. 'The Heart of the Matter' by Peter J. Mead in Arden W. Mead, *Christ is the Heart of Christmas: Devotions as Christmas Approaches* (Creative Communications for the Parish, 1980).

3. Gordon MacDonald, *Ordering Your Private World* (Highland, 1984), pp. 75–76.

4. Will Glennon, *Best Things Fathers Do: Ideas and Advice from Real World Dads* (Conari Press, 2008), pp. 17–18.

5. The National Childbirth Trust (NCT) is the largest parenting charity in the UK. For more information, see www.nct.org.uk

## Chapter 3

1. Heather Best is quoted in Jack Canfield, Mark Victor Hansen and Patty Aubery, *Chicken Soup for the New Mother's Soul: Touching Stories about the Miracles of Motherhood* (Vermilion, 2008), p. 16.
2. Vicki Iovine, *The Best Friends' Guide to Pregnancy: Or Everything the Doctor Won't Tell You* (Bloomsbury, 1997), p. 61.
3. Will and his friend Dr Rob Waller co-founded Mind and Soul (www.mindandsoul.info), a non-profit-making organization that resources Christians to explore the relationship between Christianity and mental and emotional health. The first Mind and Soul conference took place in 2008.
4. Diaphragmatic hernias occur when the abdominal contents herniate into the chest.
5. Naomi Starkey, *Good Enough Mother: God at Work in the Challenge of Parenting* (Bible Reading Fellowship, 2009), p. 65.
6. Francis and Judith MacNutt, *Praying for Your Unborn Child* (Hodder and Stoughton, 1988), p. 3.
7. You can find further practical tools to help combat worries at www.mindandsoul.info
8. See Numbers 12:5–7 and Genesis 41.

## Chapter 4

1. Lindsay and Mark Melluish, *Family Time* (Kingsway, 1999), p. 22.
2. The Parenting Course was launched through Holy Trinity Brompton. See www.htb.org.uk/parenting
3. Rachel Waddilove, *The Baby Book: How to Enjoy Year One* (Lion Hudson, 2006), p. 174.
4. Nicky and Sila Lee, *The Parenting Book* (Alpha International, 2009), p. 32.
5. Naomi Stadlen, *What Mothers Do: Especially When it Looks Like Nothing* (Piatkus, 2004), p. 213.

**Chapter 5**

1. Danny Silk, *Loving Our Kids on Purpose: Making a Heart-to-Heart Connection* (Destiny Image, 2008), p. 74.
2. Gilly Smith, *Nigella Lawson: A Biography* (Andre Deutsch, 2006), p. 24.
3. Ibid., p. 25.
4. Read the story of Hezekiah in 2 Kings 18.

**Chapter 6**

1. 'Baca' means 'weeping', 'misery' or 'tears'.
2. Article in the *Sunday Telegraph* by Laura Donnelly, 15 November 2009.

**Chapter 7**

1. A TENS (transcutaneous electrical nerve stimulation) machine applies electrical current through the skin for pain control.

**Chapter 8**

1. Naomi Stadlen, *What Mothers Do: Especially When It Looks Like Nothing* (Piatkus, 2004), p. 39.
2. Danny Silk, *Loving Our Kids on Purpose: Making a Heart-to-Heart Connection* (Destiny Image, 2008), p. 90.
3. Glenn and Natalie Williams, *Your Relationship Can Survive a Newborn* (Focus on the Family International, 2004), p. 54.
4. We recommend reading and discussing the following: Sue Palmer, *Toxic Childhood: How the Modern World is Damaging Our Children and What We Can Do about It* (Orion Books, 2007), Chapter 6, 'Who's looking after the children?' There are also some helpful comments on the issue of whether or not to work when you have a young family in Jane Bullivant, *Dear Lord, I Feel Like a Whale* (Monarch, 2004), pp. 109–111 and Nicky and Sila Lee, *The Parenting Book* (Alpha, 2009), pp. 43–46.

5. There is a short chapter on money during pregnancy and early parenthood in Glenn and Natalie Williams, *Your Relationship Can Survive a Newborn* (Focus on the Family International, 2004), pp. 35–41. For further reading on money management we recommend Rob Parsons, *The Money Secret* (Hodder and Stoughton, 2005), and a book by Ash Carter (IVP, forthcoming). We also found a useful free budget planner spreadsheet at www.moneysavingexpert.com

6. According to a survey conducted by www.bounty.com in 2009.

7. Sheila Bridge, *Who Stole Your Sex Life? Be Free from the Influences that Inhibit You* (Kingsway, 2007), pp. 163–164.

8. Cognitive Behavioural Therapy (CBT) is a form of psychotherapeutic treatment that provides an understanding of the thoughts and feelings that shape behaviour.

9. See Genesis 37.

10. See Genesis 45:4.

**Chapter 9**

1. Stacie Cockrell, Cathy O'Neill and Julia Stone, *Babyproofing Your Marriage: How to Laugh More, Argue Less and Communicate Better as Your Family Grows* (HarperCollins, 2007), pp. 17–18.

2. Ibid., p. 14.

3. From *The Oxford Dictionary of Quotations* edited by Elizabeth Knowles (Oxford Universiy Press, 2009).

4. Stormie Omartian, *The Power of a Praying Parent* (Kingsway, 1995), p. 29.

5. For more on the gift of tongues, see Acts 2:4–8 and 1 Corinthians 12:10.

6. Sila Lee, feature on Parenting in the UK, *Christianity* magazine, September 2009, p. 50.

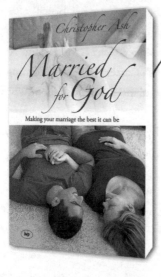

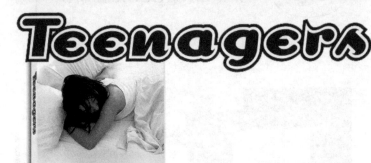

# Ann Benton

## Biblical wisdom for parents

*'Under that hoodie, behind that eye make-up, there frequently lurks a human being of immense charm, affection and wit.'*

Ann Benton admits that, when her children were teenagers, she enjoyed 'the very best of parenting years'. Yet, from her experience and that of others, she is all too well aware of the frustrations, pitfalls and difficulties that parenting teens can bring.

The Bible book of Proverbs points to wisdom as the key to health, happiness and prosperity. The author points out that the job of parents is not first and foremost to make their teens successful, but to make them wise.

With honesty and wit, Ann shows how Proverbs can speak directly into real life, however messy, today.

ISBN:
978-1-84474-354-4

Available from your local Christian bookshop or via our website at www.ivpbooks.com

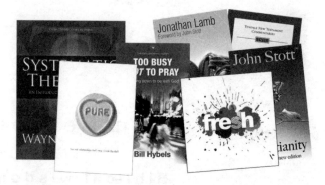